THE WILDERNESS SHALL BLOSSOM LIKE THE *Rose*

CULTIVATING
A PROSPEROUS BODY, MIND,
AND SPIRIT

THE WILDERNESS SHALL BLOSSOM LIKE THE *Rose*

FORSHIA ROSS

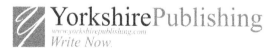

ISBN: 978-1-946977-78-6
The Wilderness Shall Blossom like the Rose
Copyright © 2013 by Forshia Ross

All rights reserved.

No part of this publication may be reproduced, distributed, or transmitted in any form or by any means, including photocopying, recording, or other electronic or mechanical methods, without the prior written permission of the publisher, except in the case of brief quotations embodied in critical reviews and certain other noncommercial uses permitted by copyright law.

All scripture quotations, unless otherwise indicated, are taken from the *Holy Bible, New International Version®*, NIV®. Copyright © 1973, 1978, 1984 by Biblica, Inc.™ Used by permission of Zondervan. All rights reserved worldwide. www.zondervan.com

Scripture quotations marked (AMP) are taken from the *Amplified Bible*, Copyright © 1954, 1958, 1962, 1964, 1965, 1987 by The Lockman Foundation. Used by permission.

Scripture quotations marked (KJV) are taken from the *Holy Bible, King James Version*, Cambridge, 1769. Used by permission. All rights reserved.

Scripture quotations marked (TLB) are taken from *The Living Bible* / Kenneth N. Taylor: Tyndale House, © Copyright 1997, 1971 by Tyndale House Publishers, Inc. Used by permission. All rights reserved.

For permission requests, write to the publisher at the address below.

Yorkshire Publishing
3207 South Norwood Avenue
Tulsa, Oklahoma 74135
www.YorkshirePublishing.com
918.394.2665

DEDICATION

To all those who thought they could never overcome the adversities of life, I dedicate this book to you. To all those who are on the very brink of giving up, I dedicate this book to you. To all those who wondered why their path was so painful and so difficult, I dedicate this book to you. And with a grateful heart, I thank my Creator for the grace He extended to me in bringing me through to the other side.

TABLE OF CONTENTS

Preface 9
Introduction 11
Prologue 15
I Will Heal You 19
A Future Promise 23
Do You Really Want Me to Go? 29
The Root of It All 35
The Imprinting of the Father 41
Bittersweet Surrender 49
God Was There All the Time 55
Meeting Eric 63
A Trip to the Commissary 73
A Hallmark Moment 83
A Painful Lesson 91
A Tabernacle in the Wilderness 101

A Spirit of Infirmity 111
A Spirit of Poverty 121
What about My Children? 131
Roses, Roses, Everywhere Roses 143
Epilogue 153

PREFACE

*H*indsight is always 20/20 as they say. Well, I'm no different, and I know you aren't either. If we were to take the time to look back over our lives and peer behind the scenes, we would discover a mysterious plan etching its way through the landscape of our lives. The adversities of life can be cruel at times, and yet it is the very fuel that can energize us to succeed. With God, this is possible. With God, our life can have meaning and purpose as our own story unfolds before those around us. As you read my story, my prayer is that it will become the fuel you need to overcome every obstacle in your life—fuel to encourage you to go the extra mile in order to reach the very best. We all have a story to tell. Every person's path is different, and yet God's principles remain the same, timeless jewels when applied in the wilderness of life. This is as it should be. This is the way the Lord planned it. We fight, we scratch, we cry, and yet in the end, if we follow our Creator, He leads us to our promised land.

As I've gotten older and, I hope, age more gracefully, success has defined itself in a richer way. Isn't that always the way of it? Yet, we all have to discover this path of inner peace and purpose for ourselves. Thank God, he didn't let me find it any other way because his ways are the best—enduring and not only affecting this short time we have here on earth but lasting throughout all eternity.

Come along with me in the next step of my journey to wholeness. You will laugh, you might even cry, and you will probably get angry at times as my story challenges you. But in the end, you will see the mighty hand of God reaching down and whispering to this servant, "Come follow me. I am the way, the truth, and the life." And in this, dear one, my hope is that you will follow God as he says to you, "Come follow me."

This is my story, this is my song—praising my Savior all the day long.

INTRODUCTION

I must say that I wish with all of my heart that I could wave a magic wand over your life and change everything that's unpleasant in an instant. That would be the way I would do it. But God has a process that we all go through to arrive at our destination. Some journeys are longer than others, and some journeys are more painful than others. But God has provided us with the promise of his word to navigate us successfully through the wildernesses of our life. This was clearly demonstrated when the Holy Spirit led Jesus into his wilderness. Satan wanted him to do it another way by twisting the true meaning of the word of his Father. But Jesus saw through his scheme and resisted, thereby overcoming the temptation to take the easy road.

In the midst of the Israelites' journey through the wilderness, God gave them a promise—a glimpse of an abundant land. And what a glimpse it was! A land flowing with milk and honey and grapes as big as apples. The only problem was that they wanted to get there in their own way. They wanted it handed to them! But

God had a better way. He knew the influence of the Egyptian world from which they had become enslaved was still part of their thinking. He knew that in order for them to fully master, enjoy, and maintain the promised land awaiting them, they would have to deal with the attitudes of their heart. They would have to learn that God was their first source. I believe the wilderness is simply a visual picture of our own heart. And God will purposefully and patiently invade it because he knows what it will take for each one of us to realize our future. The influences of our past and our own propensity to repeat it has to be *weeded* out. This process takes time as we unlearn, relearn, and yield to our loving Father. This is a good thing, but often painful.

In the midst of my painful wilderness, God gave me a promise—a glimpse of a better life—an abundant life. And what a promise it was! One morning, during a very difficult time in my life when I was seeking the Lord, I literally cried out to him for an answer. As I was reading my Bible, Deuteronomy 28:1–14 seemed to leap off the page at me. These scriptures listed all the wonderful promises God was going to do for the Israelites. I felt the Lord was also giving me these same scriptures. As I read and reread these scriptures, hope began to rise in my heart. However, as time passed, I began to see that the emphasis in this portion of Scripture was conditional. All the promises flowed from the one condition of hearing and obeying the voice of God in verse one.

And so I set out on a journey to learn how to hear God's voice and put into practice the things necessary to reap my promised land. I was to learn time and time again as the years rolled by that God's love and grace for me are always unconditional, but to enter and experience the promises were not. The kingdom of God is a realm where God ruled, not me. It is a place where his Word ruled, not what I perceive it to be. If I want to fully receive all God has planned for me to have, I have to choose his way. Did Jesus not say,

> But seek (aim at and strive after) first of all His kingdom and His righteousness (His way of doing and being right), and then all these things taken together will be given you besides.
>
> Matthew 6:33 (AMP)

In the book of Isaiah chapter 35, the Prophet Isaiah explains how the desert will come alive again, blossoming like the rose, and how the wilderness will rejoice greatly and shout with joy. Because of this, he says to strengthen the weak hands and make firm the feeble knees. He goes on to say that waters shall break forth in the wilderness and streams in the desert. The burning sand and mirage shall become a pool, and the thirsty ground springs of water. The eyes of the blind shall be opened, and the ears of the deaf shall be unstopped. The lame shall leap like a hart, and the tongue of the dumb shall sing for joy. And a highway shall be there, and a way, and it shall be called the Way of Holiness—it shall be for the redeemed. That's me! That's you!

Do you need a promise in your wilderness? Ask for one. Has God given you a promise? You must not succumb to the easy way out thereby short-circuiting your expected end. You must not quit. You must listen and yield at all costs to his voice because it is your cool drink of water in the desert. You must not listen to well-meaning friends who think surely God wouldn't ask this of you. The cost may prove high, but God's rewards will be astronomical. His love and guidance will not fail you—ever. Now I can say that my eyes have been opened, and my ears have been unstopped. I can leap like a hart, and my tongue can praise him. I can say with certainty that he *is* the pool in the wilderness that never runs dry. He is the highway—the Way of Holiness!

PROLOGUE

Wayne drove down the dirt road looking for a place to pull over. It was early in the morning. The sun had just risen and was hanging oppressively over the landscape. Alabama was so hot and steamy in July. Sometimes there was a respite from the heat early in the morning just before the sun would rise, but it would not last for long. Already I was beginning to be covered with a fine dew of sweat and feeling sticky. Pulling over at the first sight of a side road, Wayne parked, turned off the engine, and leaned back in his seat. I sat quietly, looking straight ahead, feeling a little uneasy but not knowing why. Wayne was a mysterious sort. I never could seem to figure him out and never felt secure in his next move. His conversations with me always veiled hidden motives, so I never knew what to expect.

Finally breaking the stillness, Wayne leaned over to my side of the car and reached for the glove compartment. Unlatching the door, he placed his hand inside and pulled out a gun. I sat perfectly still, trying not to act startled. As he started to talk, he turned the gun over and over in his hands. His voice was sarcastic as usual, but this time there was an unmistakable edge of depression in it—an unmistakable edge of hopelessness. I remained calm and began to talk slowly and steadily, keeping my voice low and unemotional. I don't remember anything that I said, but it must have appeased him for he placed the gun on the dashboard, leaned back, and listened. I could feel the crisis ebbing. By now, my jeans were soaked with sweat and felt heavy against my body. Rivets trickled down my temples and neck. Slowly, he picked up the gun and placed it back in the glove compartment. The crisis was over, and so was the marriage. Within a few weeks, Wayne would abandon my daughter Tiffany and me. I remember hugging her tightly as she rocked in her little rocking chair the night after he left and exclaiming as tears rolled down my cheek, "Don't worry, Tiffany. I will take care of you." She was only two.

I was only sixteen when a pattern began to emerge in my relationships with men. Here I was—after spending hours getting dressed, attending to every detail, sitting alone on my bed—waiting. Waiting had begun to be a common ingredient in our dating. Waiting for Wayne to call me, waiting for Wayne to pick me up for a date—waiting for him to give me some sign that he truly cared. He was late quite often, but this time he didn't show up at all. I was devastated. It confirmed the feelings that I quite never knew where I stood with him. Yet I pursued him. I couldn't imagine life without him. My feelings overwhelmed any *signals* that this relationship was not a healthy one.

"Forshia," called my mother. As I ran down the stairs from my bedroom to answer her, she thrust out her closed hand and then slowly opened it. There in the palm of her hand was a small diamond engagement ring. "Wayne left this for you," she said.

Ignoring her displeasure at how he had obviously asked me to marry him, I placed it on my left ring finger and jumped for joy. *Finally*, I thought. *Finally it has happened.* I had waited two years. *Finally, we're going to be married.* I was thrilled beyond belief.

We married in the summer of 1968. I was only eighteen. *The Graduate* with Dustin Hoffman was playing at the time. We were all humming the title song, "Mrs. Robinson." I hummed a lot because I was happy and ready to be a wife, keep the house, and learn how to cook. I only knew how to cook desserts. My first meal: split hotdogs with cheese tucked into the slits on a bed of rice. I was proud of my creation. How short-lived this happiness would be. In less than two weeks, the pattern of waiting would start again.

Wayne didn't show up for dinner one evening. In fact, he didn't come home that night at all. I was frantic. *Maybe he's been in an accident.* We had no phone. I had no family in the area. Though we had moved near his family, I did not know them that well as yet. As time went on, his absences would increase, sometimes for days at a time. Sometimes he would not show up for the holiday dinner I would cook. It became quite evident that I had married an alcoholic. He was cruel and mean when he drank. By then, I was pregnant with our daughter, Tiffany, and left alone most of the time. My heart was broken.

The song "Mrs. Robinson" that I hummed so often told of Jesus's love for me and that heaven was waiting for me. Did he? Did he love me? I didn't know at the time that one day Jesus would love me more than I would know. It would take many years of life-threatening twists and turns before I knew that heaven held a place for me.

I WILL HEAL YOU

*T*he vision was vivid. I saw in my mind's eye my own face broken into hundreds of puzzle pieces. The pieces were floating in the air, and then they gradually came together until my face was whole again. As my face came together, it shone with a brilliant light, so bright that it almost blinded my eyes. The vision stayed with me for weeks, and the soft inner voice of the Lord kept saying, "I am the one who will heal you. Trust me."

Walking out of the psychiatrist's office this particular day was one of the hardest things I had ever done. I wouldn't be coming back. I had told the doctor so with confidence and resolve. I had just finished my two years of preventative medicine against the mental breakdown I had had several years before. I had expressed to him that I wanted to be off of all medicines, and he had suggested that I continue on them for two years as a measure against any further breakdowns. The two years were up. He did not take the news well, and he told me so quite bluntly. "You are doing the wrong thing. I cannot give you my blessing," he said.

As I left his office, I was shaking as my confidence ebbed. Had I heard it right? Did I really see the vision? Would I ever be well? The Lord's voice was so tender at that moment. How could his voice be so tender and soft, almost as faint as a whisper, and yet powerful enough to impart to me the knowledge that I had indeed heard him correctly? "I am the one who will heal you. Trust Me," he said again. I was about to embark on an uncharted journey of monumental proportions.

The Bible tells us that the Israelites took an uncharted journey, and what a journey it was! It began with God plucking Moses out of the backside of the desert, speaking to him from a burning bush and commanding him to deliver the Israelites who were in bondage to Pharaoh in Egypt. They had been slaves for 400 years. Through miraculous signs and wonders, God did amazing things through Moses to show Pharaoh that he was God and there was no other. "Let my people go!" was Moses' constant mantra. God would have the final say and the Israelites would be set free by his mighty hand. Determined to reclaim his bounty, Pharaoh chased the Israelites to the Red Sea.

God's parting of the Red Sea so that the Israelites could cross over still astounds us today. It is the stuff of which movies are made. Crossing over on dry ground, the Israelites were finally safe from Pharaoh's clutches. Their deliverer, whom they had been promised for 400 years, had finally brought them through, Pharaoh and all his soldiers drowning as the Red Sea swept over them. Great celebration ensued with dancing and shouting proclaiming God's mighty deliverance. What a deliverance it was! I am sure, as they turned to watch their tormentors drown in front of their eyes, they did not anticipate that their ongoing journey would be long. Yet their journey to the Promised Land would turn out to be a slow and arduous one.

I didn't know it at the time, but my journey to wholeness was going to be a long one. I would discover through the years that even in a long, sometimes tedious, journey, God had a plan. His plan would take me from one victory to the next, though to the outside observer, the victories weren't always visible. What God had in mind for me would be to start from the inside out. He wanted to start with my heart. I would learn that the story of the Israelites' journey through the wilderness would mirror mine on so many levels. The only difference being that I was going to reach my promised land as Joshua and Caleb did. And yet the lessons learned from the ones who didn't cross over into the promised land would be food for fodder for all those who would heed.

In the book of Hebrews, the writer warns us not to ignore the plight of the Israelites and not to repeat their mistakes. I surmised that if the warning was there, then that meant it was possible for me to make it through. Don't get me wrong, there were more times than I can count when I wanted to give up. It was too hard at times and too long. Yet God had a unique plan for me to finish my course. As he helped me discover it, progression, though slow, continually happened. His words would be a comfort to me when I felt I had nothing left in me that would keep me going. In Isaiah 42:3, the Word of God says that a bruised reed he will not break or a smoldering wick he will not snuff out. I would discover time and again that there was always just enough flame to keep me going. I would discover no matter how bruised I felt, I would not break. I would discover he was always faithful.

I had hope. I had a vision. I was still here. I heard his voice, "I am the one who will heal you. Trust me." The Bible says in Psalm 37:23 that the Lord orders the steps of a good man. Even when my steps appeared to make no sense, my steps were being ordered. That's a comforting thought, now isn't it?

> These things happened to them as examples and were written down as warnings for us, on whom the fulfillment of the ages has come.
>
> 1 Corinthians 10:11

A FUTURE PROMISE

I fell crumpled in a heap in front of the couch. It was hopeless, I thought. I will never be like those women. They were beautiful, confident, and radiant with the presence of the Lord. My sobs were coming from a deep place of failure within me. The sobs were more than just sounds of a frustrated woman but were the sounds of a wounded animal. I cried deeply.

All of a sudden, I sensed that I should look up. The couch was in front of a bay window. It had been a gloomy day and the sky was speckled with clouds. I lifted my head just in time to see the sun escape from behind one of the clouds. A bright beam of light exploded down through the bay window and right on the bowl of fruit that was sitting on the ledge. I had made this bowl in the mental ward. "Forshia," the Lord said, "do you see the fruit in the bowl that you made in the mental ward? One day, you too will be full of fruits."

I had been attending the neighborhood Kay Arthur Bible study for quite some time. It was held in Fairfax, Virginia, where my family and I lived. Kay Arthur is a nationally known Bible teacher who had created inductive Bible studies that were taught in home groups facilitated by others. She actually came to the study one time to meet us. We were all thrilled. I loved the study, and the women who came were very loving, accepting, and always encouraging. But often I would leave the study feeling defeated. They were so beautiful and peaceful. I was depressed most of the time, overweight, and terribly unhappy. I wanted to be like them. I wanted to be like Jesus. I didn't want to be like me.

We were studying the book of Romans in the New Testament. I was truly fascinated when we came to Romans 7 where Paul explains so thoroughly how mixed up he was about wanting to do the right things and yet at the same time, he would do the wrong things. Wow! It sounded like me. Paul says, "We know that the law is spiritual; but I am unspiritual, sold as a slave to sin. I do not understand what I do. For what I want to do I do not do, but what I hate I do" (Romans 7:14–15).

How did he know I was reading my own story? And how did he get out of it? I was caught in the middle of some kind of spiritual battle. At times, I really felt that there was a dark, unseen force in the mix. The more I tried to do the right thing, the more I couldn't. It was tearing me apart. I was perplexed and at odds with myself all the time. What was the answer to this dilemma I was in? Is there an answer?

As we continued to study the chapter and come to the end, I was again confused by Paul's answer. "What a wretched man I am! Who will rescue me from this body of death? Thanks be to God—through Jesus Christ our Lord!" (Romans 7:24–25a). I could surely identify with the "wretched" part. I felt like I was back to square one before I had received Jesus as my Lord and Savior. At that time, I was struggling with being a good wife and mother. Now flashes of my terrible attitudes were showing up again. It was like starting all over.

When I received Jesus that fateful day at my kitchen table in 1978 in Oklahoma City, God flooded me with his love, which I began to shower on my family. It was as if who I really wanted to be was restored to me. It was an incredible time. But once I began to crumble emotionally and was taken to the mental ward, I struggled continually with trying to get my footing again. The more I tried, the more I failed. The more I failed, the more I felt condemned. The more I felt condemned, the more I felt hopeless. The more I felt hopeless, the more I felt depressed. I would get up each morning and try to do better, only to fail again. I had made such a mess of my life in the past and now I couldn't even get it right for God. I felt like a total failure. The condemnation was oppressive.

"Thanks be to God through Jesus Christ our Lord!" I had no recourse but to go back to this verse time and time again. I would read it and read it and read it. Only it didn't seem to help because I was still the same. "So then, I myself in my mind am a slave to God's law, but in the sinful nature a slave to the law of sin" (Romans

7:25b). It actually made so much sense. In my mind, I desired to do the right thing. Didn't I try every day? But this other part of me did right opposite. I would open my mouth to say a kind word, and out would come this other person. But I still kept going back and reading the last verse in Romans 7, "So then, I myself in my mind am a slave to God's law, but in the sinful nature a slave to the law of sin." I kept looking for the key that would connect this last verse to the answer. Only I couldn't seem to find it.

Then one day, there it was. I saw it. The answer! I had read the first verses in Romans 8 time and time again, but it never connected. I always felt like something was missing between the last verses of Romans 7 and the first and second verse of Romans 8. Funny, I kept trying to read between the lines as if God was hiding something from me. "Therefore, there is now no condemnation for those who are in Christ Jesus, because through Christ Jesus the law of the Spirit of life set me free from the law of sin and death."

The word *now* jumped out at me. There is no condemnation *now*. Not later, after I crossed all my *t*'s and dotted all my *i*'s. Some days I could, some days I couldn't. Not later, after I grunted and strained and cried out to the Lord and asked forgiveness for what seemed like a thousand times. No, it was *now*! It was now as I was doing what I didn't want to do. Why? Because I had no power in myself to do what I felt was required of me—simple things, like being nice to my family; simple things, like forgiving myself quickly when I wasn't nice. I was not condemned because I couldn't get it right. I went back to the verse in Romans 7:25b again, "So then, I myself in my mind am a slave to God's law, but in the sinful nature a slave to the law of sin."

In my mind I wanted to obey God's requirements. I wanted to please him, but alas, I couldn't, no matter how much I tried. My sinful nature always won. But even while it was going on, I was not condemned. I saw that feeling guilty and condemned actually gave sin its power. The more I couldn't meet God's standards, the more I felt guilty; the more I felt guilty, the more I felt condemned. The more I felt condemned, the more I felt hopeless. I found myself often thinking like Paul, "What a wretched woman I am! Who will rescue me from this body of death?" Thanks be to God through Jesus Christ our Lord! I began to see that the living law of Christ's spirit within me would set me free from the demands that the sinful nature within me required. Wow! This was deep and yet so simple. I began to see that each time I failed, I didn't have to feel condemned. I began to see a light at the end of the tunnel.

> And the Holy Spirit testifies that this is so, for he has said, "This is the agreement I will make with the people of Israel, though they broke their first agreement: I will write my laws into their minds so that they will always know my will, and I will put my laws in their hearts so that they will want to obey them."
>
> Hebrews 10:15–16 (TLB)

DO YOU REALLY WANT ME TO GO?

I woke up startled from a deep sleep and sat straight up in bed. Something wasn't right. I felt an eerie presence in the room and darkness darker than the room itself surrounded me. Fearful, I called out to the Lord. "What is this?" Suddenly I saw an odd-looking creature standing at the foot of my bed looking at me. It was purple and had a kangaroo-type body with a long tail. It had an almost cartoon appearance, and yet the evil that clung to it was suffocating. "Lord, what is this?" I asked.

"It is a spirit of condemnation," the Lord answered.

"What do I do?" I asked frantically.

"Just point to it and say, in the name of Jesus, I command you to go," the Lord said. With shaking fingers, I pointed to it and commanded it to go.

Its head was small, and its ears were big. With menacing eyes, it turned slowly toward me and spoke. "Do you really want me to go?" Trembling, but without hesitation, I emphatically said yes. Immediately, it tucked its tail between its legs and left with speed like lightning.

I was leaning over the bathroom sink, washing my face, pondering why I still couldn't stop struggling so much when I faintly heard in my spirit the word *condemnation*. Even though I was beginning to understand through our weekly Bible study that there was no condemnation through Jesus Christ, I still felt a powerful oppression of guilt and judgment come over me at times. And when it did come, I didn't have the strength to shoo it away. I was still struggling to do the right things and to say the right things. The dark unseen force that I had thought was in the mix was about to pay me a visit. I went to bed that night pondering all of these things. If I had known what would take place, I would not have gone to bed at all. If I had known that this would be part of the key to my freedom, I would have thought of another way.

More times than not, the Israelites wanted another way to reach the promised land. The wilderness wasn't a bed of roses that was for sure. It was a dry, hot, and lifeless land. Water was scarce, food was scarce, and the journey was monotonous. God always provided for them, but their appreciation of the provision was short-lived. They grew impatient. They wanted to go back to Egypt many times. They wanted God's provision and deliverance another way. They were getting sick of manna, sick of obstacles, sick, sick, sick of it all, and they told God and Moses so. "Why have you brought us up out of Egypt to die in the desert? There is no bread! There is no water! And we detest this miserable food!" (Numbers 21:5)

The Israelites and Egyptians had a great fear of snakes. The desert of Sinai was fret with poisonous ones. Responding to their railing, the Lord released the snakes and they bit the people, and many of them died. Repentant for complaining, they went to Moses and said, "We sinned when we spoke against the Lord and against you. Pray that the Lord will take the snakes away from us" (Numbers 21:7).

Moses prayed for the people. Now I would think that the Lord would take the snakes away after they confessed, but not so. His way of deliverance was most interesting and profound. He asked Moses to make a snake out of bronze and put it up on a pole. Then he told Moses to tell the people that if anyone was bitten and looked at the bronze snake, he would live. What a strange solution. The very thing that they were asking to be removed was the very thing they had to confront.

The Israelites would rather have had God remove the snakes altogether. I would rather have had God just deal with the demonic spirit standing before me. Couldn't I go back to sleep and pull the covers over my head? I didn't want to look at this hideous creature at the foot of my bed and feel its overwhelming evilness. Wasn't there an easier way? But I was learning a principle that would test me time and time again as I was being taken step by step into my promised land. God's solution to each obstacle in my life would be different from what I would have orchestrated. I would have to face my giants, face my enemies, and face my problems head-on. In so doing, I would learn the most important principle of my life. God had the answers, and if I looked to him for direction, he would show me what to do each time.

Yes, what a strange solution the Lord provided for the Israelites dilemma. The word from God was that when a snake bit anyone they were to look at the bronze snake on the pole, and then they would live. The Amplified translation puts it this way, "And Moses made a serpent of bronze and put it on a pole, and if a serpent had bitten any man, when he looked to the serpent of bronze (attentively, expectantly, with a steady and absorbing gaze), he lived" (Numbers 21:9 AMP). What God was asking them to do was to look to him for deliverance. The snake on the pole was lifeless, unable to harm them. Even though they were bitten, when they looked away from their pain, they were putting their trust in God's Words alone. The snakes were under God's control. The culprit of their problems was not their enemy. Complaining and impatience and yearning for another way out—that was their enemy.

"Do you really want me to go?" the demonic thing asked me. What a strange question, and yet it wasn't so strange. For the minutest of a split second, I was aware that there was an unhealthy desire in me to just let things be. It would be easier not to face this. It was more comfortable not to have to do anything. Let me snuggle back under the covers and pretend this is all a dream. In a way, I had adjusted to my oppression. It always passed if I just hung on.

THE WILDERNESS SHALL BLOSSOM LIKE THE ROSE

How sick the human nature is without the prodding of God's spirit. How often the Israelites wanted to go back to Egypt. After all, they were fed and they were clothed on a consistent basis. Makes no sense to us, and yet we are not so different without the Lord. This thing called life requires a response, and the Lord who is so infinitely patient and wondrously loving would encourage a right response every time.

No matter how long the journey was going to take, I was to learn time and time again that God's way is the most lasting and complete. Each bend in the road, each stop, each failure has a corresponding solution and victory that comes from God and God alone. He would use people, he would use circumstances, and he would use unusual solutions. But most of all he always uses the undergirding of his Word, the Bible. I would be faced again and again with a crossroads of sorts. Would I trust him? Would I seek his way? Would I yield? As weak and powerless as I was, when I did as the Lord instructed, even the powers that be would obey my command. I was amazed!

> Just as Moses lifted up the snake in the desert, so the Son of Man must be lifted up, that everyone who believes in him may have eternal life.
>
> John 3:14–15

THE ROOT OF IT ALL

*W*e were all sitting around the kitchen table. My son, my daughter, and my husband Eric were chattering away. I made spaghetti for dinner, and we were all enjoying it. My recipe was different from everyone else's, and it had become a family favorite. All of a sudden, Eric said something critical that sparked a furnace inside of me to heat up. I felt this boiling anger begin to overtake me. *That's it! I've had it!* I thought. *I won't take this anymore. I am going to take this plate of spaghetti and dump it right on his head. See if that doesn't show him.* All of a sudden, as I was struggling with the overwhelming desire to do just that, I looked at him in astonishment and blinked. His face had turned into my father's face for just a split second. I blinked tightly and looked at him again. Sure enough, my father's face was transposed over his face. Then it disappeared. It was 1983, a year I'll never forget.

I never felt secure growing up. I knew my father loved me, but over the years, I would learn that his love was conditional. I could never disagree or voice my thoughts in his presence without it turning into a major power play. I would have to stand for hours and listen as he lectured me. It was tormenting. Sometimes I couldn't take it anymore and I would rebel but he always won and his strong will always overpowered mine. Sometimes physical punishment was used to prove a point. Sometimes punishment would include shaming me in public. He would always feel bad afterward and say he was sorry. His regret was always sincere and I always forgave him. Kids do that. But around thirteen something died inside of me. I didn't love him anymore. I always felt guilty about that.

I don't think I could have voiced it then or defined it, but a deep unconscious root of insecurity and self doubt would take hold of me and plague me for most of my life. Quite often out of anger, my father would punish me, and I wouldn't know the reason. This type of punishment would even transfer into discipline from my teachers and later into adult relationships. More times than I can count, I would be confused with what I knew was true and what I was told was true. I was never allowed to make my own decisions. My father made them for me whether I liked them or not.

Somewhere deep inside me, I began to believe everyone else was right without even knowing why. Since I didn't have confidence in my own abilities, I let others script my life for me. Affirmation would become my drug of choice. This need would lead me into major life changing destructive choices based on that need. Just tell me you love me, and I'll follow you. Just give me attention, and I'll believe you. Just pay attention to me and I'll hand my life over to you. Just ask me to marry you and I will. Two abusive marriages would fail around this insatiable desire to be loved and accepted. It's a modern-day story as old as Adam and Eve and as fresh as yours and mine. Now my present marriage, my third marriage, was in trouble too. I wasn't exactly sure why I responded the way I did.

I'm sure the Israelites weren't exactly sure why they reacted like they did. Why they wanted to go back to Egypt time and time again. Their savior had come. Their prayers had been answered. God sent their deliverer just as they had been told he would. For 400 years, the story had been passed down from generation to generation. Finally the day had come. The Bible says that they left with Egypt's spoils and not one was sick among them. Their Egyptian neighbors handed over their silver and gold just for the asking because of the great fear of Jehovah God that had settled over the land. But their rejoicing over leaving lasted for only a short burst of time. All they could see was that having been delivered from Egypt, they were now facing another dilemma, another problem, with the Egyptian army hot on their trail. Why, it wasn't much better than staying in Egypt. In fact, it seemed worse. Here they were with Moses as their leader, standing before the Red Sea with no way to cross over. A cry went up from their lips.

> They said to Moses, "Was it because there were no graves in Egypt that you brought us

> to the desert to die? What have you done to us by bringing us out of Egypt? Didn't we say to you in Egypt, 'Leave us alone; let us serve the Egyptians'? It would have been better for us to serve the Egyptians than to die in the desert!"
>
> Exodus 14:11–12

Interesting. Even bondage can have its own twisted rewards, a security of sorts that requires no change. But God had another plan—a plan of deliverance. The only problem was their deliverance didn't come quite like they had envisioned. Using Moses as their leader, God pushed his people forward and faithfully answered their cry. Moses said,

> "Do not be afraid. Stand firm and you will see the deliverance the LORD will bring you today. The Egyptians you see today you will never see again. The LORD will fight for you; you need only to be still."
>
> Exodus 14:13–14

Even in the midst of their fear and doubt, God's faithfulness to his people displayed a God of love, power, and might. He would not only deliver them once, but many times, as he parted the Red Sea and ushered them through onto dry ground.

I am sure that the Israelites did not understand that the effects of being under Egypt's rule would influence their journey into the wilderness. Their hearts and minds had been affected by the years of slavery. As contrary situations arose, the conditioning of their thinking would threaten to draw them back to what they thought was the security of Egypt. Each time God delivered the Israelites, their rejoicing would last but for a short burst of time. Just like the Israelites, my past would threaten to dictate what my future would be. Just like the Israelites, it would be easier for me to resort to past behavior I had learned and react badly. I so *wanted* to dump the spaghetti on my husband's head.

As my family continued to talk around the dinner table, oblivious to my unfolding drama, I became aware of this deeper issue with my father. An understanding began to emerge. It wasn't my husband that was the problem. It was my learned perceptions and reactions based on my earthly father. That was the root of my problem. As time went on, I would discover that the effects of my childhood would play a major role in my need for emotional healing.

The Bible says that God led the Israelites by a cloud by day and a pillar of fire by night. This manifestation of his presence provided protection and direction. As God showed his patience and faithfulness to Israel, so his tender and loving presence would guide me by day, and in the thick of the night, I would learn to yield to his delivering voice. So many times, the Lord's gentle words would come back to me, "I am the one who will heal you. Trust me."

When I had asked Jesus several years earlier before this incident to come into my heart, I later was baptized. Going under the water and coming up signified the death, burial, and resurrection of Jesus Christ. It was explained to me that this was also a declaration of the death, burial, and resurrection of my life. As God sought to be Israel's leader through Moses, leading them through the Red Sea, he would seek to lead me through Jesus Christ. Each time I yielded to his way, my past would be buried and new life would spring forth—his life in me. It was time to unlearn what I had learned. It was time to bury my past. The spaghetti stayed put and I marveled at God's unfolding journey for me.

> For we must never forget, dear brothers, what happened to our people in the wilderness long ago. God guided them by sending a cloud that moved along ahead of them; and he brought them all safely through the waters of the Red Sea. This might be called their "baptism"—baptized both in sea and cloud!—as followers of Moses—their commitment to him as their leader. And by a miracle God sent them food to eat and water to drink there in the desert; they drank the water that Christ gave them.
>
> 1 Corinthians 10:1–4a (TLB)

THE IMPRINTING OF THE FATHER

The words my father and grandmother flung at each other were horrendous. It went on for hours. No curse words, just terribly destructive critical words. As they tore each other down in the kitchen, my mother would softly and quietly tuck us three kids in the one bed in the other room. I cried softly. I didn't understand why they hated each other so much. I was probably around eight. It always happened that when we got ready to leave the next morning, there would be tears, apologies, and regrets from my grandmother and my father. They were sincere as they hugged each other and told each other how much they loved each other. Without my knowing it, these incidents would leave an imprint on my heart that would carry into my adult life.

In the Merriam Webster Dictionary, the word *imprint* means "to mark by or as if by pressure," "to fix indelibly or permanently (as on the memory)," or "to subject to or induce by imprinting."

My grandmother lived in a very tiny two-room house—a kitchen and a bedroom. She was my father's mother. We called her Big Mamaw because she was big so that we could distinguish her from my maternal grandmother who was small. When we could, we would visit her because my father was an enlisted man in the Army and we moved around a lot. She lived in Clanton. That's where I was born, where my father was born, and my mother too. My sister was also born there. Clanton, Alabama was a small town about forty miles north of Montgomery.

Over the years, I would hear bits and pieces about my grandmother, things like she was an alcoholic at one time and my father had to get himself off to school every morning, how he only had water and cornflakes for breakfast, how he had no shoes because they were poor, how there were hints of other men. My grandfather eventually divorced my grandmother and married another woman. My father also tells how he wandered around the neighborhood as a small boy crying because he couldn't find his mother. It became obvious to me that his father favored his stepchildren. One time though, I saw my grandfather chase my stepaunt with a big metal chain and beat her as she ran out of the house and wrapped herself around the front porch column. I didn't know what she had done. But I loved my grandfather. He was always kind to me and always gave me a quarter whenever I saw him. Over the years, I saw my father yearn for his father's love. When my grandfather died, he left my father five dollars in his will. It broke my father's heart.

THE WILDERNESS SHALL BLOSSOM LIKE THE ROSE

As I grew up, the effects of my father's own childhood dysfunction would take on a pattern that would live itself out in our household. The fighting would take on a rhythm similar to that of the fights that my father had with his mother. Only I didn't know it had a rhythm at the time. Somehow, the whole household would become embroiled in the fights. I didn't always know exactly what they were all about or how they got started. My mother was usually quiet, always trying to calm my father down. She was often a mediator. As I grew up and time went on, the influence of this dysfunction created a behavior in me that continued the dysfunction and caused destruction in my life. It was the only way I knew how to get what I wanted or thought I needed.

My fights with Eric were just as horrendous as my father's with his mother. I actually would pick the fights, but subconsciously, I didn't know I was doing it. I couldn't seem to help it. I was good at getting my way and very rebellious. I wasn't always sure how the arguments got started, but they would go on for hours, ending with apologies, hugs and kisses, and especially regrets. I remember one time specifically when my husband expressed to me that I had caused him to question his own mind. Believe me, my husband has a brilliant mind. One day, the Lord showed me that these fights occurred about every six weeks like clockwork. I was a bit amazed until he flashed back the fights my family had had while I was growing up. Indeed, they occurred about every six weeks. I hadn't even realized that. The

Lord was beginning to unfold the imprinting influence one generation has on another.

Lack in one's life causes many things. Lack of emotional and physical needs in my life caused me to seek fulfillment using the only tools I knew. I think we are all like that to one degree or another. God created us to seek fulfillment in him. If these needs are not met, we seek them in other things or in other people. What was missing in my life created a void in me that I would try to fill long after becoming a Christian. I didn't know that these *things* I would try to get by *unlawful means* were gods—gods that took first place in my heart.

As I learned about my mother's side of the family, similar imprinting issues ensued. Her father left the family when she was fourteen and married another woman. Her grandfather was an alcoholic and often abused the family. She tells of how her grandmother had to take the children and sleep in the woods because of the drunken rages her grandfather went through. She also tells of how the KKK burned a cross in their yard, warning him to straighten up. I was told that at one time, my grandfather was a very wealthy lumber baron but lost it all due to drinking. Though my mother remained married and committed to my father and committed to our family throughout my father's life, I would experience two divorces and a string of destructive relationships before my third marriage to Eric. Oh, the imprinting from one generation to another!

God addressed the importance of one generation's influence on another as the Israelites continued their journey through the desert. In the third month after they left Egypt, they came to the foot of Mount Sinai. There the Lord called Moses from the mountain and gave him his instructions for the people. He was to consecrate the people in preparation for the third day when God would speak to them. When he did, God gave Moses the Ten Commandments that the people of Israel were to live by, the first one being, "You shall have no other god's before me." The Israelites had had many gods in Egypt and were still hanging on to them. These gods took their affection and attention away from the God who delivered them out of Egypt—the One True God. He knew in order to be able to bless and prosper them and lead them to the promised land, they would have to lay their idols down. The second commandment given by God is a most amazing one.

> You shall not make for yourself an idol in the form of anything in heaven above or on the earth beneath or in the waters below. You shall not bow down to them or worship them; for I, the Lord your God, am a jealous God, punishing the children for the sin of the fathers to the third and fourth generation of those who hate me, but showing love to a thousand generations of those who love me and keep my commandments.
>
> Deuteronomy 5:8–10

I had many idols from my past that were taking my affection and attention away from serving the One True God. These occupied my heart. Granted they were not statues like the Israelites worshipped. They were anger, bitterness, resentment, my hatred for men, manipulation to get my way, rebellion and the list could go on and on. You can add your own. Though I had legitimate painful reasons why they were there, nevertheless, these gods were controlling me. I blamed my past and everyone around me. I was not happy. I needed healing. The imprinting my father received from his father was simply being passed on to me. My father was imperfect. His father was imperfect. I was imperfect.

What was the answer? The answer was that now I had a perfect father that I could count on. The One True God I could come to know through Jesus Christ! He would show me a better way. As I trusted him and yielded to his ways, his love would break this cycle. My new Father was the heavenly Father who showed me his perfect love by sending his son, Jesus Christ to earth to die in my grandmother's place, my father's place and my place. For all those who receive this sacrifice, they would find a better way to live and interact with loved ones. This new interaction would break destructive family cycles and leave a new legacy for their children and their children's children. His love would be shown to a thousand generations to those who loved him.

Why, this new interaction could start with me! If those who hurt me did not receive this great love so that they could be healed, it did not prevent me from receiving my healing. I didn't have to keep yearning that my earthly father would finally get it right so I could be at peace. I couldn't keep blaming him for my unhappiness. No, Jesus got it right, and he could help me be the person I so wanted to be.

THE WILDERNESS SHALL BLOSSOM LIKE THE ROSE

Was this going to be easy? I dare say it was not! It would take some time to learn about this new love that my new heavenly Father had for me. It would take some time to learn I didn't have to react to others based on what others did to me. I would learn that I could trust my heavenly Father because he wanted the best for me. I didn't want to stay like I was. I wanted to change. I wanted to leave an imprint on this earth. Not a greasy spot in the road of life that people stepped around and ignored. No, I wanted to be a glorious pool of clear water that could reflect the Lord's countenance. That's what I wanted. I wanted to be like him. Whatever it took, I wanted it. Let the healing begin.

> For the law was given through Moses; grace and truth came through Jesus Christ. No one has ever seen God, but God the One and Only, who is at the Father's side, has made him known.
>
> John 1:17–18

BITTERSWEET SURRENDER

*J*put the covers over my head as if God couldn't see me. I can't possibly do what he was asking. Eric had hurt me too much. How was it right to just let him off the hook? It wasn't right. The pain was searing as the Lord brought back to me what he had done and how I needed to forgive him. It just wasn't right. What about my rights? What about my pain? Isn't God going to do something about that? Doesn't he care? I was bitter and angry. No answer. Just silence. Yet the silence was pregnant with the answer. I saw in my mind's eye the cross before me and Jesus nailed to the cross. I heard him say, "Father, forgive them for they know not what they do." I knew there was no other way. There was no turning back.

The struggle was intense. It would take me two weeks to make the decision to forgive my husband. And it *was* a decision. It surely was not based on my feelings about the whole thing. My feelings wanted acknowledgement. My feelings wanted revenge hidden in so many passive-aggressive ways. My feelings were all over the place. I wrestled with the fact that my husband might never acknowledge what he did. I wrestled with the fact that if I forgave him the way Jesus forgives, I could not throw it in his face again. The matter would have to stay dead and buried. No strings attached. Boy, did I know about strings. My love had countless strings. My love was conditional. I knew what God was asking of me, and it hurt. It hurt real bad. I wrestled with the knowledge that God was asking me to obey him without knowing the outcome of my obedience. He was my example in living and, if need be, in dying also. I *had* agreed to follow him.

After the joyful celebration of crossing the Red Sea, it didn't take long before the Israelites were unhappy again. Following Moses into the desert, they were like unruly children fighting against anything that didn't go right. For three days, they traveled in the desert of Shur without any water until they came to Marah. But the water there was bitter. So the people grumbled against Moses, saying, "What are we to drink?" (Exodus 15:24) When Moses cried out to the Lord, the Lord showed him a piece of wood. He threw it into the water, and the water became sweet. Here is a wonderful picture of God's intended provision for the Israelites. Even though they grumbled, God had a plan of redemption right in the middle of their *bitter experience*. The piece of wood would make the water sweet. The Lord was showing them that if they obeyed his voice, he could and would make things better. I dare say that the piece of wood that Moses threw into the bitter waters pointed to the cross of Jesus Christ. His ultimate sacrifice was my example. I would learn that if I heeded the voice of the Lord, the miracle I was looking for was right under my nose. All that Jesus accomplished on the cross could happen right in the middle of my circumstance. The answer wasn't somewhere else. The miracle was waiting on me. Forgiveness started with me.

This encounter at Marah set a precedent for the Israelites that would instruct them on how they were to respond to the Lord. The Bible goes on to say that at the waters of Marah, the Lord made a decree and a law for them and there he *tested* them. I believe the adherence to these instructions would determine the length of time they would wander in the desert. It didn't mean they would never be tested again, but the response to the test could determine whether they would stay where they were or move on to greener pastures. Listen to the Lord's promise.

> He said, "If you listen carefully to the voice of the LORD your God and do what is right in his eyes, if you pay attention to his commands and keep all his decrees, I will not bring on you any of the diseases I brought on the Egyptians, for I am the LORD, who heals you."
>
> Exodus 15:26

"I am the Lord who heals you." Similar words that were spoken to me by the Lord when I left the psychiatrist's office: "I am the one who will heal you. Trust me." In my pursuit of healing, learning to listen to his voice and obey him would become my most ardent quest and the Bible my greatest teacher. Hidden in the pages of the greatest book ever written would be the answers I needed. The Kay Arthur Bible study I attended each week was a bright spot in my life. It was my lifeline to hope. I could hardly wait until the day rolled around. Though I continued to struggle with depression and sometimes felt overwhelmed by the study, I learned some invaluable truths that would become part of my study habits. These truths would set the stage in helping me learn how to walk through difficult places in my life.

The greatest truth would be that the Bible *is* true and that I could *hear* the voice of the Lord through the scriptures. I could rationalize, cry, kick, scream, and hurt like crazy, but in the end, Jesus had the word of life and the Bible was still true. Did he love me in my pain? Absolutely! Did he identify with my pain! Unequivocally! Did he hate the injustice? Yes, the Bible teaches that he does! He accomplished all of this on the cross when he said, "It is finished," in John 19:30. But I'm talking about going on to greener pastures. Remember? I'm talking about being healed, walking in peace, and being like Jesus. Egypt is a place of defeat. The promised land is a place of victory!

I forgave my husband, and the peace came. In fact, the Lord took all of the pain when I did. I no longer hurt. I was healed. To this day, I don't remember what my husband did. I'm pretty sure it was a conglomeration of things that had piled up in the early part of our marriage. This can be so common in marriages. I would also have to go to Eric and ask for his forgiveness—forgiveness for venting my frustration out on him for what had happened to me in my past. I often used him as a scapegoat for my unhealed heart. We hurt each other a lot in the beginning of our marriage, but through forgiveness, healing came. In Matthew 6:14–15, Jesus says, "For if you forgive men when they sin against you, your heavenly Father will also forgive you. But if you do not forgive men their sins, your Father will not forgive your sins."

Forgiveness is a powerful thing. I shudder to think of what the future might have been if I had not learned to forgive. My bitterness would have grown. It would have poisoned all those who came in contact with me. The Bible teaches us in Hebrews 12:15, "See to it that no one misses the grace of God and that no bitter root grows up to cause trouble and defile many." This encounter with the Lord set a precedent for my future because I would have many opportunities to forgive in all kinds of situations. Don't get me wrong. Sometimes it would take me a few days to make the decision. But if you can conquer this one, you can make big leaps and strides across the desert. Can't you see it? The promised land, that is!

> So, as the Holy Spirit says: "Today, if you hear his voice, do not harden your hearts as you did in the rebellion, during the time of testing in the desert, where your fathers tested and tried me and for forty years saw what I did.
>
> Hebrews 3:7–9

GOD WAS THERE ALL THE TIME

I cried out to Bill in the middle of the night. The pain was horrific. I knew I needed to go to the emergency room. I tried to awaken him, but he kept going back to sleep. Finally, in a panic, I screamed at him, trying to get him to listen.

With one swift kick with his foot, he sent me tumbling onto the floor. "Now leave me alone, and let me get some sleep," he said, irritated. He was a big man—six foot two and weighed 250 pounds, all muscle and bone. I was no match for him.

Crawling to the bathroom, I pulled myself up using the commode as leverage. I was having problems standing. Looking into the mirror, I gasped. My face looked like a monster. Huge welts the size of small plates contorted my face. The pain in my feet was worse. I gasped again. My feet were almost twice their size, and my toes were completely black. I crawled to the couch, crying, and curling up in a ball, I waited until morning. We lived in the country. We had no phone, and I had no money.

I met Bill at the Top of the Stars. It was a nightclub on the top floor of the Holiday Inn in Montgomery, Alabama. Bill asked me to dance, and we began dating soon after. My daughter Tiffany and I lived with my parents at that time. I had been divorced from my first husband, Wayne, for about two years. I had a good job, a brand-new car, and had bought some new furniture. My plan was to eventually move out of my parents' house so I could be on my own. Though by most standards my life was modest, I was still proud of how far I had come since the divorce.

It wasn't long before Bill asked me to marry him, but I had begun to feel uneasy about the relationship, so I turned him down. But Bill was a very convincing man. I knew he loved me, and he proceeded to tell me how much. I knew he loved Tiffany, perhaps more than her own father, showing her care and attention that he had not. But I couldn't seem to resist anyone who expressed a need for me. As always, I struggled with trusting my own perceptions. I was so easily swayed. I said yes and married Bill. It was around 1972.

The pattern of abandonment that I had experienced with Wayne began almost immediately. Bill took me to Mobile, Alabama, where he was from, for our honeymoon, dropped me off at some friend's house early in the day, and didn't show up until late that night. Bill was an ex-convict and supposedly a reformed drug addict. I knew this when I married him. How naive I was. As I look back, it was obvious that he was out scoring drugs as I sat waiting for him. This marriage would plunge me into a nightmare and a seedy side of life that I thought I would never escape from. From the Top of the Stars to the bottom of hell, I would sink into an abyss of gargantuan proportions, taking my daughter with me.

Bill took me to the county hospital that morning and dropped me off. The doctors could not find the root cause for the swelling in my face and feet but attributed it to stress. Stress! Are you kidding me? No one knew the stress I was under. Looking back, I believe the stress was so intense my body rebelled. I kept our situation from my family and friends, mainly because I didn't want to admit I had made another mistake. I didn't want to hear my father tell me, "I told you so."

I kept trying to make the marriage work. I was the only one contributing to the household finances. Bill couldn't keep a job and when he did have one, he spent it on drugs. There was not enough food most of the time, not enough gas to go to work most of the time—not enough of anything. Sometimes, I would drop him off at work when he did get a job, only to find out it was all a setup. There was no job. There would be somebody waiting for him around the corner to pick him up for a day of drug deals.

The marriage took me from a modest form of stability to living on the top floor of a condemned rat-infested house with no heat and no hope and holes in the floor. I remember standing at the bottom of the stairs of this house one day. I was sweeping the stairs, trying to bring some order to our hovel. I wanted a home. I wanted order. I cried softly at how pitiful my attempt to bring order was. The sorrow was too deep for words. Suddenly I *felt* a dark presence at the top of the stairs. I sensed it moving toward me. I didn't know it at the time, but this encounter with darkness would play a major role in my need for healing in the future.

> The LORD said, "I have indeed seen the misery of my people in Egypt. I have heard them crying out because of their slave drivers, and I am concerned about their suffering. So I have come down to rescue them from the hand of the Egyptians and to bring them up out of that land into a good and spacious land, a land flowing with milk and honey…"
>
> Exodus 3:7–8

The Lord saw and was deeply moved by what the Israelites were going through. He was there all along, and he had a detailed plan to deliver them from Egypt and lead them out of where they were. Why were they in bondage for so long—400 years? Why did God allow them to go through what they went through? That, I don't know. I do know his intentions were not only to rescue the Israelites but also to prosper them. I did not know God then in the way that I do now. I didn't even seek him during that time. I felt I had to figure it out all by myself.

Yet he was watching over me, and he felt my grief. He was there all along. "For we have not an high priest which cannot be touched with the feeling of our infirmities; but was in all points tempted like as we are, yet without sin" (Hebrews 4:15, KJV). Jesus felt what I was feeling, and he was helping me. How did I know this? I didn't know it at the time, but as I look back, I remember the check that showed up in the mail from the government just when I needed it. It was a check that had apparently been owed me for many years.

I remember the time Bill was so impaired on drugs and alcohol that he lost control of the car while we were driving home on the freeway in Montgomery. We spun around three times, missing a transfer truck by a hair, just in time for me to look up into the driver of the cab and catch a glimpse of the red glow of the cigarette hanging from his mouth. I was so hysterical when we came to a stop that Bill had to slap me. I can still see the driver standing on the side of the road shaking like a leaf, waiting to see if we were all right. My life was spared that night because God was there. He was watching over me. He had a future plan for me.

I remember walking the streets with Tiffany after Bill didn't pay the rent at one place we lived. When I found this out, I told Bill not to come home. I had had enough. In fact, it would be the last time I would see him until our divorce. The landlady said we had to be out by the following Monday even though I begged her to understand that it wasn't my fault that Bill had not paid the rent. She would not listen. I took Tiffany's hand and just started walking the streets, not knowing what I was going to do or where I was going. After walking for a while, I saw a sign Room for Rent in the window of an old house. I only had thirty-five dollars. I asked the landlord if he would trust me with the rest when I got paid. I told him I had nowhere else to stay. He let me move in. You see, God was there all along, behind the scenes, moving on this man's heart to help me.

I remember having an abscessed tooth and no money to go to the dentist. One side of my face swelled up, and even though the pain was unbearable, I still had to work. Someone told someone who asked a dentist to look at me. He fixed my tooth and only charged me a minimal fee. You see, God was there! I remember time and time again Bill pressuring me to put the needle in my vein. He was a powerfully convincing man, and yet I wouldn't do it. Yes, I did drugs too—liquor, pot, Quaaludes, speed, even LSD once. But I wouldn't mainline. I had heard that once you do that, there is no hope of ever being free of it. But it was really God giving me the strength to resist. He was there all along.

The Bible teaches in Hebrews 13:8 that "Jesus Christ is the same yesterday and today and forever." Jesus was in my yesterday, even though I didn't know it. He didn't *cause* my yesterday, but he was there. He was helping me though I could not *see* him. He was concerned about my sufferings. Even though my choices had put me there, he took pity on my frame. Even then, his spirit was warning me not to marry Bill. He still understood my weaknesses, even my rebellion. He didn't even judge me!

In John 3:17, we read that God did not send his Son into the world to condemn the world, but to save the world through him. The Israelites chose idolatry. They mistrusted God and they rebelled time and again; yet he still loved them in their sin as he loved me. Time and again, he sought them out. Time and time again, he delivered them in their wilderness. Oh, the unfathomable love and mercy of God!

> Go, assemble the elders of Israel and say to them, "The LORD, the God of your fathers—the God of Abraham, Isaac and Jacob—appeared to me and said: I have watched over you and have seen what has been done to you in Egypt. And I have promised to bring you up out of your misery in Egypt into the land of the Canaanites, Hittites, Amorites, Perizzites, Hivites and Jebusites—a land flowing with milk and honey."
>
> Exodus 3:16–17

God would use my past in the future to help people for I understood what it was like to feel trapped, alone, and desperate. I understood what it was like to be hungry and afraid for my life. I understood what it was like to try and try and yet find that nothing worked. I understood the hopelessness and the pain of betrayal and abandonment. There would come a day when I would be able to thank the Lord for my past because it was the catalyst that would eventually lead me to him. The Bible says that those who are forgiven much love much. I would be forgiven much, oh so very much! Yes, God was there all along and he was going to use my past for his glory.

For he says to Moses, "I will have mercy on whom I have mercy, and I will have compassion on whom I have compassion." It does not, therefore, depend on man's desire or effort, but on God's mercy.

Romans 9:15–16

MEETING ERIC

I sat on the edge of the bed in the dark. I felt alone, abandoned, and ashamed. I just had an abortion. I didn't even know the father's name or where he lived. It was a one-night stand with someone I had met at a club. The effects of the abortion were unexpected. An almost tangible, overwhelming cloud of dark gloom came into the operating room when the abortion was performed. I didn't understand why I cried immediately. I felt it was my only option. I didn't know what else to do. As I sat there, I softly cried and lifted a prayer to God. I had never prayed before, and the words that escaped from my mouth were almost unintentional yet surprising. Without thinking, I said, "Would you send someone to love me?"

I met Eric at the Officer's Club at Maxwell Air Force Base in Montgomery, Alabama. He was a captain in the air force at the time and was there temporarily to go through Squadron Officer's School. He asked me to dance and then invited me over to his table. He seemed nice, but I didn't really care. I had decided to give up on men. They only brought you heartache and misery anyway. I was only there with a couple of girls because I was lonely. The abortion experience had left me empty, numb and restless.

When I asked him what he was drinking, he said, "Club Soda." *Club Soda*, I thought, *that's different*. I asked him why. He said he didn't drink much. I was immediately enthralled. After the substance abuse with my former two husbands, I had made a vow that I would never again get involved with anyone who had a problem with drugs and alcohol. I drank a couple of drinks socially, but I never really liked the stuff too much myself. It's just what you did when you went to a club. As we talked, I noticed a kindness and gentleness about him. He asked me out the next evening. When I told him I reserved Sundays to be with my daughter, Tiffany, he said to bring her along. That was different also. Most guys didn't want to be bothered with my daughter.

We dated quite a bit during the next six weeks, and as we got to know each other, I shared everything about my life, even the abortion. He was so kind and compassionate. He didn't judge me. I drank it up like a thirsty woman on a desert. Then he asked me to marry him. I had one more criteria before saying yes. "I can't marry you unless you can take care of me financially," I said. I had taken care of two husbands before, and I wasn't going to do it again. He immediately whipped out his checkbook, showing me the balance after paying the mortgage on the home he owned. My eyes got as big as saucers. I said yes!

As we settled into military life at Wright Patterson AFB in Ohio, where he was stationed before going to school in Montgomery, the real Forshia began to immerge. I didn't understand it at the time, but I had developed a *man-hating spirit*. After years of abuse at the hands of men, my reactions to his guidance and leadership in the marriage were vicious. Instead of understanding that he was trying to take care of me and protect me, I took it as another man's attempt to try to control me. I set the marriage up for failure from day one. I didn't understand my responses and couldn't seem to stop them. As I fought him tooth and nail, we began to bring out the worst in each other. The only reason I stayed was because I could not bring myself to surrender to another failure.

In a few months, Eric would be reassigned to Tinker AFB in Oklahoma City, Oklahoma. Within five months of arriving, I would become pregnant with our son, Dax. I would become increasingly unhappy, vindictive, and lost. I felt sad that my daughter Tiffany and Dax were caught in the middle of my dilemma. Tiffany had already been through so much before I married Eric in my search to fill the void in my life.

This man-hating spirit subconsciously blamed men for all of my problems. My responses to Eric were rooted in my relationship with my father and any other man I felt had hurt me. I didn't realize that God had indeed answered my prayers and had sent Eric as the man who would love me and stand by me. And he did love me. He loved me unconditionally. He was like the Rock of Gibraltar. No matter what I did or said—and I said plenty—he stayed. He wouldn't let me push him around. Even though I wanted my own way all the time, deep in my heart, I was glad he wouldn't let me. I don't think I would have respected him. I tried him to the uttermost. I was indeed a mess.

Right in the middle of my mess, God intervened and saved me. Filled with new hope, I nevertheless continued to struggle within the marriage. When Eric received orders to be stationed at Andrews AFB in Maryland and later at the Pentagon, God would unfold a plan of redemption, healing, and a course of action that would set my feet on a right path. We settled down on the outskirts of Washington, DC, in Fairfax, Virginia. Tiffany was eleven, and Dax was three.

Not too soon afterward, I would be led to the Kay Arthur Bible study facilitated by Barbara Jones where I would learn how to begin to find answers to my problems. After we went through the book of Romans, we also did a Bible study on marriage. I would learn that my ongoing grumbling, faultfinding, and rebellion against my husband was really against God. Some of the women at the Bible study had marital problems too, but they handled it differently by responding in godly ways. I was indeed convicted.

> So Moses and Aaron said to all the Israelites, "In the evening you will know that it was the Lord who brought you out of Egypt, and in the morning you will see the glory of the Lord, because he has heard your grumbling against

THE WILDERNESS SHALL BLOSSOM LIKE THE ROSE

> him. Who are we, that you should grumble against us?" Moses also said, "You will know that it was the Lord when he gives you meat to eat in the evening and all the bread you want in the morning, because he has heard your grumbling against him. Who are we? You are not grumbling against us, but against the Lord."
>
> Exodus 16:6–8

As you can see, the Israelites were unhappy again. They were grumbling because they had no meat and were comparing their life now to the life they had in Egypt. Even though they continued grumbling, God sent them an abundance of quail that covered the camp in the evening and bread from heaven in the morning. This bread was called manna. It covered the ground with thin flakes like frost that was white like coriander seed and tasted like honey. Imagine all the meat you can eat and bread supernaturally falling from heaven. Listen to God's instructions concerning the manna:

> Then the Lord said to Moses, "I will rain down bread from heaven for you. The people are to go out each day and gather enough for that day. In this way I will test them and see whether they will follow my instructions. On the sixth day they are to prepare what they bring in, and that is to be twice as much as they gather on the other days."
>
> Exodus 16:4–5

He answered their cries for meat, but with the answer came detailed instructions. Nevertheless, some of the people did not follow his instructions and tried to save some of the manna for the next day. It stunk and became full of maggots. Against God's instructions, some went out on the seventh day to gather the manna, but there was none. God's desire was to shower down his blessings upon the Israelites and meet their needs over and above. And he did. They would eat manna for forty years, and the Scriptures say that even their clothes did not wear out as they wandered through the desert.

But the Bible also says that the trip to Canaan was only an eleven-day trip. Many died along the way. Their continued disobedience to his instructions would keep them out of the promised land. Yes, God continued to meet their needs because he is a faithful God. But to enter into his greater plan would take a people sensitive to his voice—a people that would follow his instructions so that victory could be won at every turn. During this time, the Lord would give me a personal promise from the book of Deuteronomy that would set my heart to dancing:

> If you fully obey the LORD your God and carefully follow all his commands I give you today, the LORD your God will set you high above all the nations on earth. All these blessings will come upon you and accompany you if you obey the LORD your God:
> You will be blessed in the city and blessed in the country.
> The fruit of your womb will be blessed, and the crops of your land and the young of your

livestock—the calves of your herds and the lambs of your flocks.

Your basket and your kneading trough will be blessed.

You will be blessed when you come in and blessed when you go out.

The LORD will grant that the enemies who rise up against you will be defeated before you. They will come at you from one direction but flee from you in seven.

The LORD will send a blessing on your barns and on everything you put your hand to. The LORD your God will bless you in the land he is giving you.

The LORD will establish you as his holy people, as he promised you on oath, if you keep the commands of the LORD your God and walk in his ways. Then all the peoples on earth will see that you are called by the name of the LORD, and they will fear you. The LORD will grant you abundant prosperity—in the fruit of your womb, the young of your livestock and the crops of your ground—in the land he swore to your forefathers to give you.

The LORD will open the heavens, the storehouse of his bounty, to send rain on your land in season and to bless all the work of your hands. You will lend to many nations but will borrow from none. The LORD will make you the head, not the tail. If you pay attention to the commands of the LORD your God that I give you this day and carefully follow them, you will always be at the top, never at the bottom. Do not turn aside from any of the commands I give you today, to the right or to the left, following other gods and serving them.

Deuteronomy 28:1–14

The Lord spoke to me as I sat on the edge of the bed. It was a scene not so different from the time I prayed to God to send someone to love me. This time though, I was seeking to please God. I wanted to follow him. But I had pushed my husband away, and in a strange twist of fate, in some ways he was becoming just like the men I feared. I had created what I feared most.

As the Lord spoke to my heart, he made it very clear that some of my continued battle with health issues stemmed from my rebellion against my husband. He was asking me to yield to his leadership and to quit fighting him. I struggled with the request. Every fiber of my being fought against it. I was truly afraid. I reasoned that if I submitted to my husband, he would take advantage of me just like my previous husbands. I was afraid that I would disappear, that I would lose my identity. But my rebellion wasn't really against my husband—it was against God who created my identity. My identity had gotten lost. I was trying to find who I was, using my own devices, and it wasn't working.

During this time, the Lord revealed to me an amazing scripture:

> Jesus answered, "My teaching is not my own. It comes from him who sent me. If anyone chooses to do God's will, he will find out whether my

> teaching comes from God or whether I speak on my own.
>
> John 7:16–17

In other words, if I would choose to yield to God's wisdom, it would prove to be right. If it comes from God, it must be right. Sitting on the bed that day, I timidly said, "Lord, I don't think I can do this."

Immediately, the Lord's soft but firm voice came as he reminded me of the scripture in Philippians 4:13, "I can do everything through him who gives me strength." If I listened to his voice, he would make me the head, not the tail. I would always be at the top, never at the bottom.

"Yes, Lord," I replied softly.

> And don't murmur against God and his dealings with you, as some of them did, for that is why God sent his Angel to destroy them.
>
> 1 Corinthians 10:10 (TLB)

A TRIP TO THE COMMISSARY

I had promised Dax that after we finished grocery shopping at the military commissary, we would stop off at the park so he could play. I had felt pretty good that day. I still struggled with oppressive depression most of the time, but that day, my mood was light. We zipped through the commissary rather quickly, which was unusual. Civilian grocery stores were much easier to shop, but the prices were so much higher. I was a frugal shopper, yet any frustration at shopping at the commissary was usually worth the price cuts.

By the time we left the commissary though, I began to become increasingly depressed. As I sat down on the park bench to watch my son play, the darkness came in like a flood and engulfed my soul. *What happened?* I thought. *I was fine this morning. I was fine when we got to the commissary. I was fine—*

As I sat on the park bench feeling discouraged, the Lord whispered an instruction to me, "Trace your thoughts all the way back to the point at which you started feeling down."

"Okay," I answered. As I tediously retraced my thoughts all the way back to their beginning, I was amazed. At that point, a negative thought had entered my mind. I spiraled down from there. It had happened so quickly. Then the Lord asked me if the thought was true. "No, it wasn't." I realized. Immediately my mood lifted. Wow! This was amazing to me. I was on the road to something new. I was being introduced to a key to *part* of my healing from depression.

In the *World Book Dictionary*, the word *depression* means "the act of pressing down," "a sinking," "a lowering," "a hollow place," "sadness," "gloominess," "low spirits." I can add some meanings of my own. They are feelings of hopelessness, despondency, foreboding and worthlessness, insecurity, inadequacy, and low self-esteem. With these feelings came fatigue and a lack of motivation, overeating and physical problems. With all of this also came a desire to isolate myself. Can anyone relate?

Though my issues were complex, the Lord began to show me that his answers were simple. If anyone could complicate matters, I could. I thought I had to figure things out all by myself. But the Bible teaches that when we receive Jesus Christ as our Lord and Savior, we also receive his Holy Spirit within us. The Bible also teaches that the Holy Spirit is given to us, among other reasons, to guide us into *all* truth. If I listened and yielded to the Holy Spirit's guidance, he would direct me to the truth. He would direct me to the right scriptures for my situation. More often than not, he would show me the truth about myself, which wasn't always pretty. I just needed to listen and follow his direction. There was simplicity in obedience. He still loved me if I didn't listen, but I wouldn't reap the benefits of Deuteronomy 28:1–14 that he had promised me. I failed many times, too numerous to count, but I learned that he was always there to help me get back up and forge forward. It was always about my *willingness* to follow him. In Isaiah 1:19, we read, "If you are willing and obedient, you will eat the best from the land..." This simply means that it isn't just a matter of obedience, but it is also a matter of a willing heart. In the Lord's eyes, you can't have one without the other and expect things to work. I often remember my children obeying me but at the same time having a contrary attitude. It did not delight this mother's heart, though I loved them and nothing would have ever changed that. The Lord wants willing participants because he knows best. This delights his heart. He gets excited when we believe him. After all, he created us. He created me, and he knew how to fix me.

This course of action would lead me through many years of tests and trials as the Lord led me step by step in pursuit of wholeness. I would have wanted the healing process to go quicker as I know the Israelites would have wanted to reach their promised land in a shorter time. But God's ways are best, of course. In our trials, we not only discover the God that we serve, but we also find out about ourselves. Our faith is tempered, and we become strong enough to overcome anything. Yes, I would have wanted the process to be shorter, but God's ways are for a reason.

> But I will not drive them out in a single year, because the land would become desolate and the wild animals too numerous for you. Little by little I will drive them out before you, until you have increased enough to take possession of the land.
>
> Exodus 23:29–30

It wasn't always easy to do it God's way. It took time for God to work in me. Sometimes "catching" a wrong thought before it consumed me was tedious work. But I had thought wrong for so long I needed to uproot these deep-seated roots. These roots were strong in me from years of yielding to them. I needed to learn to keep doing it his way until there was lasting change in me. I needed to *wait* for God to work. I was not only developing spiritual habits by doing this, but I was also replacing the lies I had believed for so long with God's truth.

The Israelites had not done this. They had not learned to *wait* for God. They continued to buck God on every front. When Moses went up to Mount Sinai to hear from the Lord, he was given the commandments written on stone tablets by the finger of God. How awesome! But Moses was so long in coming back down that the people became impatient and asked Aaron, Moses's brother, to make them gods who will go before them. Aaron had the people bring him gold earrings that they had brought from Egypt and made an idol cast in the shape of a calf for them to worship. Listen to what they said, "These are your gods, O Israel, who brought you up out of Egypt" (Exodus 32:4b). What? This golden calf delivered them from Egypt? How deceived we can become when we don't wait for God's timing in our life. While this was going on, God spoke to Moses while he was on the mountain.

> Then the LORD said to Moses, "Go down, because your people, whom you brought up out of Egypt, have become corrupt. They have been quick to turn away from what I commanded them and have made themselves an idol cast in the shape of a calf. They have bowed down to it and sacrificed to it and have said, 'These are your gods, O Israel, who brought you up out of Egypt.'" "I have seen these people," the LORD said to Moses, "and they are a stiff-necked people."
>
> Exodus 32:7–9

My wrong thoughts had become idols—idols I worshiped. No, they weren't golden calves, but they were taking the place of God's truth. When I replaced these thoughts with truth, I became grounded, and when I thought God was late in coming down from my mountain, so to speak, I could wait and, in the waiting, not go back to relying on my past ways of thinking. I was seeing that little by little my enemies were being driven out of me. My enemies were many. Lies about myself, lies about how God wanted to work things out for my good, lies that he had a good plan in all that I was going through. If God had done all that I had wanted him to in my timing, Satan would have taken advantage of me because God wanted my cooperation. He wanted me to trust in his goodness. He wanted me to trust him step-by-step.

We read in Isaiah 28:10, "For precept must be upon precept, precept upon precept; line upon line, line upon line; here a little, and there a little" (KJV). One scripture at a time became my building blocks to healing. My emotional, mental, and physical problems were so complex that one scripture at a time was all I could handle. My Bible became my lifeline and instruction manual and the Holy Spirit my guide.

As our Kay Arthur Bible study continued to meet, I began to transfer the method of study we were learning into my daily life—my marriage, how to raise my children, and especially concerning the depression I continued to experience. The Lord would show me a scripture for each situation. I would study it and, with his help, apply it to my daily life. I was amazed as I saw results. I discovered that there were answers for each and every situation I struggled with.

The first scripture the Holy Spirit led me to in beginning my mental health was in Proverbs 3:5–6, "Trust in the Lord with all thine heart; and lean not unto thine own understanding. In all thy ways acknowledge him, and he shall direct thy paths" (KJV).

I kept a separate notebook for these personal scriptures, and using the tools learned in our Kay Arthur study, I dug deeper. *Strong's Concordance*, which is an exhaustive listing of every word in the Bible and its meanings according to the Hebrew or Greek, was our most important tool other than the Bible. The Old Testament was originally written in Hebrew and the New Testament in Greek. We would look up pertinent words in our scripture reference and write down the meanings listed in our concordance. I became fascinated with the hidden meanings of the words. It was amazing how the meanings brought greater clarity and understanding. It was like looking through a high-powered microscope and discovering the meaning of life.

Because I still suffered from depression, my study had to remain simple. For instance, we were instructed to purchase colored pencils to outline our scriptures using different colors for different word usages. It reminded me of English class in high school. I didn't like outlining sentences. I wasn't good at it. This exercise though was intended to help us in our Bible study. But I remember coming home one day and getting so confused because I couldn't decide which colored pencil to use that I broke down and cried. I felt so stupid. Depression is like that.

But the Lord gently showed me to choose one color and this would work. I still use this method today in my personal study and in teaching my Overcoming Depression Workshop. I have found that no matter how hard our life may be, God will have a plan that will work for each individual situation. He cares enough to show us even the smallest instruction that will help us. Over the years, the Lord would often whisper to me, "Forshia, keep it simple!"

We were then encouraged to consult our commentary *after* we gleaned meaning from the scriptures so that we could see that indeed the Holy Spirit had instructed us. I saw that my findings were almost always the same as the commentaries. How amazing! I didn't have to be a theologian to study the Scriptures. The Holy Spirit's job wasn't just to fill my head with knowledge but to fill my head with truth. How encouraging!

In the scripture Proverbs 3:5–6, "Trust in the LORD with all thine heart; and lean not unto thine own understanding. In all thy ways acknowledge him, and he shall direct thy paths," the word *trust* means "to hie for refuge, to be confident or sure, bold and secure." The word *heart* means "the feelings, the will, and even the intellect." It also means "the center of anything." The word *lean* means "to support one's self, to rely upon, to rest one's self, or to stay." The word *understanding* means "to separate mentally or to distinguish, to consider or to look well to." The word *ways* means "a road as trodden, a course of life or mode of action." It also means "conversation." The word *acknowledge* means "to know, observe, to recognize." In the dictionary, it means "to admit to exist or be true." The word *direct* means "to be straight or even; to make right, pleasant, and prosperous." The word *paths* means "a well-trodden road or the manner in which you go." It also means "a race." I would put it all together using the meanings from the original Hebrew language, and it went something like this:

> I can be confident and secure in the Lord. I can run to him for refuge. He is my shelter for

protection from danger or trouble. I don't have to rely on my own feelings and what they say to me. I don't have to try to figure things out with my own mind. I can even trust him with my will. In fact, I can know and recognize what his way is. I can lean into Jesus who supports me and I can stay right there in a restful state. I can be at peace as I trust him. The Lord says if I do this, he will straighten out the way I am going, which right now is a bit crooked. In fact, the way I am going right now is confusing, but he has promised if I trust him with my mind, will, and emotions, with my whole heart, he will make my path right, pleasant, and prosperous.

Every time I would get a thought that troubled me, I would apply this scripture. I didn't have to trust my own thoughts. I began to see that my thoughts or my understanding that were contrary to God's thoughts or his Word was sin. I discovered that not only does sin mean "an offense," but the root meaning of the word *sin* in the Greek language means "to miss the mark and so not share in the prize." Wow! I had missed the mark all through my life. I didn't want to miss it anymore. I wanted to win my race—my race of not letting sin be my master. I wanted to win the prize—the real prize of one day hearing the Lord say to me, "Well done, thy good and faithful servant!" As I yielded to the truth of God's Word, healing followed. Even my emotions started behaving. *Truth first equals health and wholeness later.*

Yes, steadily and ever so carefully the Lord would lead me. Step by step he would show me his truth. Step by step I would become stronger and stronger and more victorious as I allowed his truth to take root in me. Scripture by scripture, God would begin to build the foundation stones of my life—one stone upon another. Each victory brought me closer in taking possession of the promises of God. Oh, how I loved God's Word!

> One of the teachers of the law came and heard them debating. Noticing that Jesus had given them a good answer, he asked him, "Of all the commandments, which is the most important?"
>
> "The most important one," answered Jesus, "is this: 'Hear, O Israel, the Lord our God, the Lord is one. Love the Lord your God with all your heart and with all your soul and with all your mind and with all your strength.'"
>
> Mark 12:28–30

A HALLMARK MOMENT

*I*t wasn't the first time I had stood before the greeting card display not knowing what to do. The time that I dreaded was fast approaching. That time was Father's Day. Each card I picked up, I carefully put back into its slot. The words on each card expressed what a father was supposed to be. *No, that one won't work*, I thought. No, none of them were true. I was in a quandary. I had forgiven my father. The Lord had healed my heart. But what was I to do? I couldn't be a hypocrite. I felt bad.

I reached for one more card. The front of the card showed the back of a man sitting in a car driving. The rearview mirror in front of him was the focal point. The mirror was embellished with plastic to look like glass. The card said something about looking back at all the good times we experienced as father and daughter. The Lord spoke softly to my heart. "Not all of your experiences were bad. It's time to focus on the good in your past."

It was true. Not all of my experiences were bad. The card was perfect and spoke volumes. My father loved to drive and go places. He was full of surprises. Sometimes, he would wake me and my brother and sister up in the middle of the night, pile us all into the car half asleep, and off we would go to our grandmother's house. Lying in the back seat with the smell of coffee coming from my mother and father's thermos was comforting. Often, my father would look in the rearview mirror to make sure we were okay. I can still feel the gentle rocking of the car as we crossed the ferry to Mamaw's house as I was lulled back to sleep. One time, while we were staying at our grandmother's house, I remember waking up to discover that my mother and father had taken off to Nashville to see the *Grand Ole Opry* in the middle of the night. I did not realize until the mid 1990s that God was going to use these experiences to instill in me a love for travel. This love for travel would prepare me for my ministry.

There would be countless similar surprise trips over the years as I grew up. We went camping, visited relatives, and went sightseeing. I still have fond memories of stopping off at country stores to have thick slices of bologna cut for our lunch. My mother would lean back from the front seat, handing us our sandwiches. She always squished the sandwiches between her hands so the bologna would stick to the soft bread and not fall out so easily. Yes, not all of my experiences were bad. Not only would I begin to view my past differently, but I would also begin to see the frailty of human nature. Everyone had struggles. Everyone had limitations.

THE WILDERNESS SHALL BLOSSOM LIKE THE ROSE

My mother was only fifteen and my father was sixteen when they married. Theirs was a romance of which movies are made. My father saw my mother walking down the street in the tiny town of Clanton, Alabama, one day. He saw her from the window of a bus. He had just come home from a furlough with the army. He had actually lied about his age to join the army, which is impossible to do at this day and age and get away with it. He would later tell the family that my mother was so beautiful that he got off of the bus and followed her into the local drugstore/soda shop. My mother was indeed beautiful. She looked very much like Vivian Lee, who played Scarlet in *Gone with the Wind*. Then and there he asked her to marry him. He swept her off her feet, she says. They agreed to meet again at a specified time at the soda shop. She ran home and told her mother she was going to marry this man but realized that she didn't even know his name. They married in two weeks.

My mother's family owned a peach farm, so they were quite comfortable financially. She tells of her father promising to buy her a Cadillac if she didn't marry my father. But she did.

I came along three years later, then my sister and brother. Being so young, they struggled much financially. My mother tells me how she would secretly forgo the protein in the meals she cooked so my father could have a larger portion since he worked. She also tells me how, as I got a bit older, I would get nervous between meals because we didn't have quite enough food to eat. She says she felt bad about that and felt it was what contributed to my having issues with food most of my life.

As God dealt with me about focusing on the positives in my past, knowing about the struggles my parents encountered with being so young gave me a new perspective. Who was I to judge? Most of us have tried to be good parents. We have all fallen short. We all come with some baggage from our past, both big and small, that contributes to how we raise our children. We want to do the right thing, but we have all made mistakes. I surely wasn't a perfect parent. In fact, the instability of my past life was no picnic for my daughter, Tiffany. Yes, who was I to judge?

As Moses continued leading the people through the wilderness, God would descend upon Mount Sinai with fire. The whole mountain was in flames and smoke with thunder and lighting. The whole mountain shook violently and the people were afraid. The Bible says that God wanted the people to know he was serious and to pay attention. I would think so! Wouldn't you? There he issued the Ten Commandments.

> And God spoke all these words:
>
> "I am the LORD your God, who brought you out of Egypt, out of the land of slavery.
> "You shall have no other gods before me.
> "You shall not make for yourself an idol in the form of anything in heaven above or on the earth beneath or in the waters below. You shall not bow down to them or worship them; for I, the LORD your God, am a jealous God, punishing the children for the sin of the fathers to

the third and fourth generation of those who hate me, but showing love to a thousand (generations) of those who love me and keep my commandments.

"You shall not misuse the name of the Lord your God, for the Lord will not hold anyone guiltless who misuses his name.

"Remember the Sabbath day by keeping it holy. Six days you shall labor and do all your work, but the seventh day is a Sabbath to the Lord your God. On it you shall not do any work, neither you, nor your son or daughter, nor your manservant or maidservant, nor your animals, nor the alien within your gates. For in six days the Lord made the heavens and the earth, the sea, and all that is in them, but he rested on the seventh day. Therefore the Lord blessed the Sabbath day and made it holy.

"Honor your father and your mother, so that you may live long in the land the Lord your God is giving you.

"You shall not murder.

"You shall not commit adultery.

"You shall not steal.

"You shall not give false testimony against your neighbor.

"You shall not covet your neighbor's house. You shall not covet your neighbor's wife, or his manservant or maidservant, his ox or donkey, or anything that belongs to your neighbor."

Exodus 20:1–17

The fifth commandment is an interesting one. It says, "Honor your father and your mother, so that you may live long in the land the LORD your God is giving you." Here is a promise with a condition. *If* I honored my mother and father, I would live long in the promised land. In other words, I would experience a long life and continue in the place of blessing. I would continue reaping the benefits of God's good pleasure.

I would have to learn how to walk in this because my encounters with my father were volatile. I was to learn that honoring did not mean exposing myself to abuse. It did not mean accepting everything that was said to me. What it did mean was placing value on two very human beings that gave me birth, raised me to the best of their ability, and still loved me. It meant not trying to change them. It meant accepting them as God did. It meant learning how to respond differently. It meant not dancing the toxic dance that my father and I did throughout my life. With God's help, I quit arguing with my father. With God's help, I quit trying to defend myself. With God's help, I quit looking for my father's approval and affirmation. As I grew in my stability with the Lord, I also grew in my mature responses.

The last time I would see my father and mother before my father died would be one of the most pleasant visits I would ever have. I realized long after he died that this visit was a planned gift from God. During the visit, my father began to challenge me about something. I turned gently to him and said, "Dad, you know I don't do that anymore." What I meant by this was that I no longer entered into arguing with him anymore. My father loved to debate. Only he never lost.

THE WILDERNESS SHALL BLOSSOM LIKE THE ROSE

For example, if I said blue, he would say red. But then if I agreed and said red, he would go back to blue.

My father grew quiet and answered me, "Yes, I know," he said. I *had* changed, and it was evident to him. What a wonderful time we had that week. I had learned to enjoy him as he was. I know this is not always possible in some cases, but I do know that God can make a way to honor our fathers and mothers even if it is honoring them from a distance. The only way you may be able to honor your father and mother may be simply by forgiving what they have done to you. It's all a matter of a willing heart and a matter of attitude. This is honoring to God.

In the book of Hebrews 12:18–21, the author explains how now that we know God through Jesus Christ we no longer have to come to a mountain like the Israelites did. This was a mountain that displayed the awesome power of God in such a terrifying way that even Moses said, "I am trembling with fear." This was a mountain where the presence of God descended in such a way as to evoke fear from the people. No, we now have a new covenant with God. His love demonstrated through Jesus Christ would pave the way for our freedom of choice. This love is intended to evoke a desire to please God because he loves us and knows what's best for us. I choose him who speaks to me. I choose to honor.

> But you have come to Mount Zion, to the heavenly Jerusalem, the city of the living God. You have come to thousands upon thousands of angels in joyful assembly, to the church of the

firstborn, whose names are written in heaven. You have come to God, the judge of all men, to the spirits of righteous men made perfect, to Jesus the mediator of a new covenant, and to the sprinkled blood that speaks a better word than the blood of Abel. See to it that you do not refuse him who speaks.

Hebrews 12:22–25

A PAINFUL LESSON

*A*s I stood in the shower contemplating what my brother, Jay, had said, I was perplexed. I had driven down to Atlanta from Virginia to see him and his wife, Clary, and then planned to go on to Montgomery, Alabama, to see my sister, Sarita. It had been a long time since I had seen them. The night before, we had sat around visiting and reminiscing about our lives. One thing led to another, and before we knew it, Jay and I were talking about the struggles we had had with our father. I rehashed all the painful instances, my brother having some of his own.

When our conversation drew to a close, my brother turned to me and said questioningly, "I thought you said you had forgiven Dad?"

I have, I thought. But I couldn't argue with his question. After all, I didn't sound like I had.

I turned to the Lord. "Have I, Lord?" I asked. "I thought I had."

The answer was simple but profound. "Yes, you have, Forshia, but your spoken words are not backing up that truth."

The cold sores were painful. I had them all over my mouth. Not just one or two or even a few, but they surrounded my lips. I had been struggling with them for months. I must have tried every ointment on the market. I was embarrassed, to say the least. The antibiotic ointment the doctor had given me wasn't working either. The cold sores continued. Finally, I asked the Lord about it. I was still learning to seek the Lord about everything. In my personal Bible study, I discovered that Jesus didn't do anything without first hearing from his heavenly Father. This fascinated me. I surmised that if Jesus had to consult his Father on everything, how much more would I need to. Still, consulting the Lord on everything didn't come second nature to me.

The answer he gave me blew my socks off! I would never have imagined in my lifetime that the answer was right under my nose *literally*. The impression from the Lord was strong. "The reason, Forshia, you are afflicted with these cold sores is because you have a critical mouth. It's not because I am afflicting you, but the power of your words are creating this affliction."

Wow! I was utterly amazed. I *did* have a critical mouth. It was true. I only knew how to find fault or disapprove. I only focused on what was wrong, not on what was right. I only saw the negative not the positive. My critical mouth was creating negative results. How could my husband learn about God's love through me? I was a frustrated woman whose mouth gave her away. How could my brother or anyone else know the awesome forgiveness of Christ unless my actions supported my change of heart? I was a terrible witness, not necessarily to those in my Bible study or my church, but to those that counted most—my family. Woe unto me!

Family was the hardest. The closeness of family brought out stuff in me I needed to deal with. My husband didn't even know it, but God was using him to make me more like Christ. It was painful at times to hear what came out of my mouth. Ugh! Help me, Lord. Even my children, as sweet as they were, were being used to show me where my priorities really were. I was a self-centered person. With all of my heart, I wanted to be a Christ-centered person. I had a lot of learning to do about the ways of God.

During this time, the Lord had me look up the word *frustrate* in the dictionary. It means "to make an effort seem useless, thus keeping a person from doing what he wants or has set out to do." That was exactly how I felt. I felt like no matter what I tried to do or say, my efforts ended in frustration. I couldn't get the results I wanted or the responses I needed, so I resorted to coercion. God's ways are so different. He did not browbeat people to get what he wanted even if they were wrong. He did not want me to resort to coercion when I was frustrated or manipulate situations. He wanted me to trust him having faith that in due season He would work things out.

> What is faith? It is the confident assurance that something we want is going to happen. It is the

certainty that what we hope for is waiting for us, even though we cannot see it up ahead.

Hebrews 11:1 (TLB)

He wanted my interaction with others to be positive displaying the hope and patience that God extends. No one likes to be pushed into a corner. I know I didn't. His perspective is so different. He saw what I could be. He saw what others could be. He saw what my family could be. He had a good plan in mind.

It became obvious to me that the root of my frustration stemmed from not really knowing that God wanted the best for me. He wanted me to succeed. He cared about my hopes and dreams. Not all of my desires were wrong; I was just going about it in all the wrong ways. Listen to what God says in Jeremiah 29:11, "For I know the plans I have for you," declares the LORD, "plans to prosper you and not to harm you, plans to give you hope and a future." Yes, he had a good outcome in store for me. *I didn't have to get my way in the wrong way.* I could learn to be the way God intended me to be—a woman of hope, grace, and faith, a woman who could draw forth the best in people with God-filled wise words. I sure had a lot of *unlearning* to do. I wrote the scripture on a card and put it on my desk. I read it often.

From the beginning, God showed us his ways. Even after Adam and Eve sinned by eating from the tree of the knowledge of good and evil, God did not turn his back on them. He still wanted to fellowship with them. He did not give up on them. Their sin of disobedience did not keep God from providing a solution for their failure. It was the same with the Israelites in the desert. God consistently appealed to their heart, desiring that they would trust in his ways. He proved time and time again that he would move in their behalf. He had a plan. His plan was to take them somewhere—somewhere that was better than where they had been, somewhere that was better than where they were. They had trouble believing this so they complained and grumbled and found fault with God and Moses. They had trouble waiting to get *there*.

In Psalm 103:7, the Bible says that God made known his ways to Moses, but his acts to the children of Israel. I wanted to know God's ways, not just his rescues. He picked me up every time I failed, but I wanted more than that. I wanted to know his ways, so that I didn't have to fail all the time. I didn't want to have to reap the bitter fruit of my ways. I wanted to display the fruit of God's ways—his spirit was love, joy, peace, patience, kindness, goodness, faithfulness, gentleness, and self-control as expressed in Galatians 5:22. This was God's way. He wanted my words to express this fruit. In this was creative power.

In the first chapter of the book of Genesis, God spoke our world into existence by using words. His very first words were, "Let there be light," and the Bible says that there was light. He simply spoke it, and it was. When he had finished, he said everything he had created was very good. After God created Adam and Eve, he placed them in the Garden of Eden and told them that they could eat of any tree in the garden but not the tree of the knowledge of good and evil. Then that old serpent, the devil, came and tempted Adam and Eve to disobey God. The rest is definitely history. Sin came into the world. Darkness came into the world, and mankind has since struggled with not only obeying God's ways but also understanding them.

God's ways always shed light on a problem. He said let there be light! He even created the moon and the stars to shed light in the darkness. In Proverbs 18:21, the Bible states that life and death are in the power of the tongue and those who love it will eat its fruit. I was reaping the creative power of my tongue. My critical words were not creating a place for hope to be expressed. My words were creating a death of sorts. Proverbs also says that the tongue that brings healing is a tree of life.

We know that Adam and Eve ate from the tree of the knowledge of good and evil. Their eyes were opened to evil, and the battle between light and darkness has been ongoing every since. But God sent his son, Jesus, into the world just at the right time to solve this problem. By receiving his son into our very core—our heart of hearts—his light floods our soul with truth. As we receive and walk in this truth, our lives will change, and we will bring hope to others. Think about it. When you turn on a light switch in a dark room, the light chases the darkness away.

> In the beginning was the Word, and the Word was with God, and the Word was God. He was with God in the beginning. Through him all

things were made; without him nothing was made that has been made. In him was life, and that life was the light of men. The light shines in the darkness, but the darkness has not understood it.

John 1:1–5

"Even the darkness will not be dark to you; the night will shine like the day, for darkness is as light to you" (Psalm 139:12). What this means to me is that no situation is too dark that God can't bring his light into. *What shall I do, Lord? How do I change my wicked ways?* My words were creating destruction not just to those around me but also to myself. I consistently spoke ill of myself. I would tell myself that I couldn't do anything right, often looking into the mirror in my bathroom and repeating my thoughts of how ugly I thought I was and how stupid I felt. I was reaping the words of my own mouth. I wanted to understand his ways.

The first step to my healing was an interesting one. The first thing the Lord led me to do was to go on a fast for thirty days.

"Thirty days! I had never gone on a fast before." I was still a rather young Christian. "Wouldn't thirty days without food kill me?"

The Lord spoke again. "I don't want you to go thirty days without food. I want you to go thirty days without saying anything critical."

I realized that being critical had become a stronghold in my life. Fasting would break this stronghold. It was the hardest fast I would ever go on. As I starved myself from critical, negative, and condemning words, it was obvious how strong this stronghold was. I could barely watch television without seeing something negative even in how a person dressed. I didn't do the fast perfectly, but by the end of the thirty days, the power of this sin's direction in my life was broken. Now as I relied on the Lord, he would help me change the way I spoke.

Just as God spoke our world into existence with words, my words had creative power. This was an incredible revelation from the Lord. How God created the heavens and the earth showed us his ways. The result of his words was *very good*. I would learn that my words could set the stage for God to work something good in my life, my family's life, and others by what I said. The results of my words could be *very good*. Did that mean I didn't acknowledge the problems in my life or address them? Did that mean I looked at things through rose-colored glasses? Did that mean I stuck my head in the sand like the proverbial ostrich? No, it didn't. What it did mean was that I would be able to look beyond the problem with an expectation of hope. It meant that what I saw was not necessarily the final curtain call. It meant I could focus on the positive things that took place each day in my life. It meant that I could focus on the positive characteristics of my husband. It meant that the promises in the Word of God have the final say.

Another exercise the Lord showed me to do to help me change my focus and my way of thinking was to keep a journal. Each day I was to write down what I was thankful for. It was amazing how much there was to be thankful for when you looked for it. I listed all the positive qualities in my husband and thanked the Lord for them. Doing this caused me to see how God was indeed moving in my life. Why, he was there every day, all day.

I also began to find Scripture promises that would fit my particular needs. I would personalize them and then speak them *out loud* regularly. The Lord was revealing to me how powerful it was to speak his word out loud. Hearing these faith-filled words helped displace my own negative thinking. It was a wonderful life-filled cycle. For instance, in one of my earlier journals I wrote a promise from Proverbs 31 concerning my character as a wife.

> A wife of noble character who can find? She is worth far more than rubies. Her husband has full confidence in her and lacks nothing of value. She brings him good, not harm, all the days of her life.
>
> Proverbs 31:10–12

I would personalize this scripture and speak it out loud. I would say, "I am a wife of noble character. I am worth far more than rubies. My husband has full confidence in me, and my husband lacks nothing of value. I bring him good, not harm, all the days of his life." I would do this regularly. It was like prophesying my future!

I would also find promises concerning my health. I still suffered with many physical problems resulting from the side affects of the medicines I had taken from the mental breakdown. For instance, I would personalize 3 John 2 and speak out loud these words, "I pray that I may enjoy good health and that all may go well with me, even as my soul is getting along well."

I had a lot of fears, so I would personalize this scripture in 2 Timothy 1:7, "Thank you, Lord, that you have not given me a spirit of fear but a spirit of power, a spirit of love and a spirit of self-discipline." Through my Bible study, I discovered that the word *self-discipline* in the Greek also means "emotions." This was exciting to me because I craved to be emotionally stable. "Yes, I am emotionally stable," I would say out loud.

I began to experience a lift in my mood. This new focus brought a positive change in my mind and my body. I began to view things differently. My outlook began to change. This was the way of God, and it was *very good*. If I had forgiven someone, my words needed to match that truth. If I wasn't who I wanted to be yet, I could find a promise of who God said I could be! My journal became full of light, and I saw changes take place around me. Yes, sprinkled throughout my journal were still entries of struggles, pain, and many questions, but as I learned God's ways and put them into practice, his Word turned on the light switch. My thinking changed, and my outlook changed. There are approximately three thousand promises in the Bible. I had enough to last a lifetime.

> For we also have had the gospel preached to us, just as they did; but the message they heard was of no value to them, because those who heard did not combine it with faith.
>
> Hebrews 4:2

A TABERNACLE IN THE WILDERNESS

The tiny shoebox house was amazing, and so was my mother. She was an incredibly creative woman able to use whatever was at hand to turn what looked like nothing into something spectacular. It was raining that day, and I was bored. As usual, my mother would turn this day into a day to remember. Using a shoebox for a house, she made curtains from scraps of fabric and attached them to the inside of the box. Taking two pieces of cardboard and some scissors, she snipped and folded until a couch and a comfy chair seemed to appear as if by magic. The tiny Chanel No. 5 perfume box was perfect for a television set. She added knob details to the set with a pen and placed it inside in front of the couch.

She added more details to the box, and before I knew it, the little house was complete. I played with it all day as the sound of the summer rain gently danced on our tin roof. My mother always smelled of Chanel No. 5. Her fragrance and the rhythmic sound of the rain made the world a perfect place. In her presence, I always felt safe and at peace.

The ark of the covenant was a small boxlike structure made of acacia wood and was overlaid inside and out with pure gold and was about the size of a small coffee table. It would become the focal point of worship for the Israelites. The lid, which was called the mercy seat, was also covered with gold. At each end of the lid were two solid gold cherubim with wings outstretched toward the center. Inside the small box was a jar of manna, the tablets of stone on which the Ten Commandments were inscribed, and Aaron's rod that had budded. This would be the meeting place of God—the inner core of the sanctuary where his very presence rested over the cherubim. The golden altar of incense sat in front of the curtain that separated the holy place from the holy of holies. Only the high priest appointed by God could enter this room and that only once a year to atone for the sins of the people.

In building the tabernacle in the wilderness, God's instructions to Moses were explicit. Every detail down to the colors of yarn, the choice of wood, the types of metals, even the measurements and the placement of furniture were to be done exactly as the Lord had directed. This tabernacle and every detail would point to the coming Messiah. It would be a prototype of Christ himself. He would come into our midst as a *human tabernacle* able to become our sinless sacrifice for sin, our direction for life, and the place where God dwelt. No longer would a sacrifice of the blood of animals be required in order to worship God. Jesus Christ himself would become the perfect sacrifice by shedding his own blood on the cross. He would fulfill all of the requirements of the law. When Jesus died, the Bible says that the curtain that separated the holy place from the holy of holies was torn in two from top to bottom. No longer would we have to go through all the rituals as the priests did in order to meet God in the Holy of Holies. We could come boldly to the throne of grace and find mercy in times of need. He would "tabernacle" with all those who received him. He would be our dwelling place. He would invite us into his heart for he would become our true sanctuary. We could feel safe and secure as we followed his leading.

When the tabernacle was finished, a cloud covered it and the glory of the Lord filled the tabernacle. In Israel's travels, whenever the cloud lifted from above the tabernacle, they would set out on their journey, but if it did not lift, they would remain where they were.

What is most amazing are the materials God needed to construct the tabernacle were *already* available to the Israelites. Moses had asked them to take an offering for the Lord from what they *had*. They had brought much spoil from Egypt. They were to bring their silver, gold, and bronze, their colored yarns, their animal skins, olive oil and fragrant incense, and their gems, all for the construction of the tabernacle and the priest's garments. Then all of those who were skilled were to come and build his tabernacle. There were master craftsmen, designers, and weavers. Everything needed to build this tabernacle in the wilderness was right in their midst.

In the most difficult and darkest times of temptation, I would learn that everything I needed to overcome my struggles was right in my midst. Christ living in me had all the answers, all the solutions, and all the tools needed to build a godly life. Just like the tabernacle in the wilderness, everywhere I moved, Christ moved with me. *I didn't have to move alone.* When the Holy Spirit led Jesus into the wilderness to be tested and tried by Satan, he fasted forty days and forty nights and then Satan tempted him. He overcame every temptation. He overcame every temptation for us. This became a reality to me. If Christ did not succumb to Satan's temptations, then I didn't have to either. Jesus now lived in me. His presence and power was there for me. These qualities *moved* with me. His power *moved* with me.

The Israelites wandered in the wilderness for forty years. I didn't have to. I could rely on Christ's victory to overcome anything that life threw at me. I wanted to loose the weight I had gained as a side effect from the medicines I had taken. I wanted to overcome the tormenting fears that still visited me in the night seasons. I wanted to learn to love unconditionally. I wanted to be secure, strong, and stable. Sometimes, thoughts of suicide would still come crashing into my mind uninvited. But I learned that through Christ's provision, there was no temptation that could overcome me.

> No temptation has seized you except what is common to man. And God is faithful; he will not let you be tempted beyond what you can bear. But when you are tempted, he will also

provide a way out so that you can stand up under it.

1 Corinthians 10:13

His divine power has given us everything we need for life and godliness through our knowledge of him who called us by his own glory and goodness.

2 Peter 1:3

The creative side of God became very real to me. I began to look for the way God would provide so I could keep from buckling under when I was tempted. He always provided. The Bible says that he will even create a way where there seems to be no way. When finances were low and I had a need, I would become excited to see how he would provide. When I made room for God to move, his provisions came.

But it wasn't only for needs that I looked for. He also gives you the desires of your heart. Even in simple things, I saw how many of the things I wanted to do were already within my reach. Once, my son had a project due for school, only he didn't tell me until the last minute. It was too late to go to the store for the supplies, and he was so distraught at the thought of getting a bad grade that I turned to God and said, "Okay, Lord, you know what we need. What can we use that is already in the house to make this project?" I went around the house with my eyes and spiritual ears open, looking. I went down in the basement, looking. "Where is it, Lord? I'm looking." There it was—in the basement—something we would have never thought of to use for his project. This was more exciting than going to the store and buying it.

I applied this principle in everything. There was no obstacle to what God could do. As I learned more about the nature of God, I discovered that he wanted the best for me. I know I wanted the best for my children. "If you, then, though you are evil, know how to give good gifts to your children, how much more will your Father in heaven give good gifts to those who ask him!" (Matthew 7:11)

One day, as I was driving home from doing errands, I saw a chair sitting on the side of the road next to a trash barrel. I stopped and took a look at it. Surely this was a mistake. Surely the owner didn't want to throw this out. The Queen Anne–style chair had perfectly unmarred dark wooded legs. The upholstery was just as perfect with no tears, a light-green oriental-print silk. I could find nothing wrong with it except for a small stain underneath the cushion. It was obviously an expensive piece. It wasn't easy getting it into the car because of its weight, but I definitely managed. I learned that if I didn't have the money for such an expensive piece, I didn't have to settle for second best. God could provide the best.

One time, I was driving on the famous Washington, DC, Capital Beltway, making my way back home, when I heard the voice of the Lord speak softly. "Stay very still. Don't change lanes, nor speed up, or there will be an accident." The Beltway was always tricky to navigate and the traffic horrendous. I gripped the wheel tightly.

THE WILDERNESS SHALL BLOSSOM LIKE THE ROSE

All of a sudden, I was aware that several cars behind me and several coming up on both sides of me began to weave sharply all at once around me, cutting in front of my car. This went on for several minutes as cars sped up, cutting in front of me and changing lanes. They all came within inches of sideswiping my car. Just like the tabernacle in the wilderness, the Lord went with me and desired to protect me.

In Exodus 33, Moses asks God to teach him his ways so that he would know him. The Lord replied and said that his presence would go with him and he would give him rest. I loved what Moses's reply was. "If your Presence does not go with us, do not send us up from here" (Exodus 33:15). In other words, I don't want to move unless you move with me. The Bible says in Acts 17:28a, "For in him we live and move and have our being." I didn't want to move without him.

There is another creative incident with my mother when I was about six years old that I often think of with awe. It was a very hot, humid Alabama day, and we all went down to my grandmother's well where it was cooler. At the time, my family was living with my grandmother in Talladega Springs while my father was stationed in Germany for three years.

Talladega Springs, Alabama, is a small country town situated at the foot of a mountain fifteen miles from Sylacauga. Sylacauga is where the famous singer and Gomer Pyle personality, Jim Nabors, lived. Talladega Springs had one store and one bank at the time. That was about it and a railroad track that ran through the town. Once in a while, a train would go through the town, and if I happened to be there when it did, the conductor would throw out handfuls of bubble gum from the window to all the kids.

As usual, my mother had one of her creative ideas that day at the well. As I tried to stand very still, my mother carefully "sewed" leaves together on me with thorns from a nearby bush, making me a jumper. I stood very still, or at least I tried to, because every time I moved, the thorns would prick me. This took several hours.

Who would have ever thought of doing something like this except my mother? I know she missed my father terribly and made a point to keep busy. She would often call me in from playing and make me stand on a stool while she designed a dress on me. I always had to stand still, which was very hard. I was not fond of those times because I wanted to play. This incident by my grandmother's well makes me think of how often we as humans use our own ways to cover things up. It started with Adam and Eve. When they disobeyed God by eating from the tree of the knowledge of good and evil, of which they were told not to, they tried to hide and cover their nakedness with leaves. What's wrong with leaves? Nothing per se, but it wasn't God's solution to their problem.

I didn't realize it at the time, but this creative gift the Lord had given me that had been such a comfort through difficult times would also become out of balance. I loved to sew and loved fabrics. When I was unhappy, I would buy fabric. In fact, so much fabric, I had trunks full. I spent quite a bit of money to fill a void in my heart that I didn't know was there. When I was unhappy, I would neglect my family in order to sew. Yes, this gift from God was a good thing, and yet it had become a way of escape.

I had been sewing since I was ten years old. In fact, my mother handed me a needle and thread much earlier than that. I still have a small scrap of fabric with a button sewn on it and the needle I had used. My mother kept it in my baby book. All through school, I took art classes, learned to draw, watercolor, and do pottery work. Later I would learn to work in leather and woodwork. I loved crafts and putting things together. I remember one of my favorite gifts at the age of eleven for Christmas was a craft kit. When I started crafting, everything disappeared—any worries, concerns, or problems I couldn't handle. I didn't have to think about these things when I creatively worked with my hands. But just like the tabernacle in the wilderness, this gift could not be a substitute for the real thing. It couldn't remove the issues of the heart.

One day, the Lord asked me to lay down my sewing. It wasn't easy, but I had set my heart to follow him. My time would be devoted to raising my children, putting myself fully into making a home, and learning to be a godly wife.

Several years later, the Lord would give me back this gift. It would actually be sweeter than before. Isn't that the way of it? When God is in it, it is always better. He opened up a craft business for me, and I started making these beautiful life-size geese with hand-quilted wings using exquisite fabrics. I loved fabrics and had a unique gift for putting colors and prints together. These geese became very popular, and I began to get many orders. I would ask the women to trust me with picking out the fabrics. I just asked them to tell me what color they wanted. They were always thrilled with my choice.

One day, a woman who had ordered one of my geese said excitedly when she first saw it, "Why, I believe this goose is going to talk at any moment!" I knew that somehow, in a mysterious sort of way, God's presence was *with* this goose. It was giving silent glory to him.

The Bible says that Jesus's appearance didn't necessarily draw people to himself. In fact, in Isaiah 53:2, the Bible says that he had no beauty or majesty that we should be attracted to him. There was nothing in his appearance that we should want him. The skins covering the tabernacle in the wilderness were plain and unattractive, but layer by layer, this simple but profound and detailed structure revealed the beauty inside. At first glance, the instructions of his Word would seem hard to me at times, but when I yielded to his leading, a whole new world would open up. His presence and power and blessing would go with me, and he would give me peace. And best of all, I could share this "living tabernacle" with others in real ways and spread everywhere his truth like a sweet perfume.

> The point of what we are saying is this: We do have such a high priest, who sat down at the right hand of the throne of the Majesty in heaven, and who serves in the sanctuary, the true tabernacle set up by the Lord, not by man.
>
> Hebrews 8:1–2

A SPIRIT OF INFIRMITY

*A*s I lay flat on my back, I knew I was fighting for my life. My breath came in snatches. My lungs were filling up with fluid, and I felt like I was drowning. I felt as if an elephant was sitting on my chest. I was very weak, but I lifted my arms as far as I could, bending them at the elbows. Clinching my fists, I shouted with barely a whisper, "I shall not die, but live, and declare the works of the Lord" (Psalm 118:17, kjv). But at the same time, I didn't understand why this was happening. I had been free of this infirmity for quite some time. "Lord, I thought you healed me of this?"

All of a sudden, I had a vision. In my mind's eye, I saw a door. I was on one side of the door, and Satan was on the other. He had one foot on the door jam and with both hands on the doorknob; he was trying with all of his might to open the door. I could see the door slightly buckling under the strength of his pressure.

It was 1956, and Christmas was just around the corner. I was only seven years old. I had just walked up to my second grade teacher and told her I didn't feel well. She was irritated because someone in the class had just thrown up on her that day. She proceeded to tell me not to do the same and to go to the restroom quickly. I felt really strange and very weak. When I got back to my class, I laid my head on my desk barely able to move. All I remember next was lying on the couch at home. We still lived with my grandmother, and I could hear my mother and grandmother talking as if in a distance, but I could see them hovering over me. "She's delirious," my mother said. Later I would be told that I was talking a lot but not making sense. "She's burning up," she said as she began to bathe me down with cold water.

Rushing me to the hospital, I would be told later that I had almost died. I had double pneumonia. I have snatches of images in the hospital. I remember the nurses making me stand on a cold metal platform without a shirt on to take chest X-rays. It was hard to stand. I had very little strength. I remember the crushing weight on my chest when the nurses would have to remove the oxygen tent to administer medication. I remember my teacher coming to see me. I could see in her face that she felt bad for how she treated me. I remember getting Christmas presents in the hospital, especially the xylophone, which I liked.

I made a lot of noise, causing complaints from those on the floor. Apparently, there was no room for me in the children's ward when I was admitted, so they had to place me in an adult wing. The adults did not like the

THE WILDERNESS SHALL BLOSSOM LIKE THE ROSE

noise, but the nurses scolded them saying, "This little girl almost died."

I wanted to be brave when we left the hospital and refused the wheel chair, but I remembering feeling like I should let them wheel me to the car because I was so weak. Though Christmas was over by now, when I got home, my mother had saved my presents for me. They were still under the tree. As always, she made Christmas special even though it was late. It would take quite a long time for me to regain my strength and be well again.

But something strange happened from that time on. I would suffer year after year with the common cold. Only, my common cold wasn't like everyone else's. It wasn't so common. My lungs would seem to fill up with mucus, and the cold would last for months during the winter seasons. I would cough until I was exhausted trying to clear my lungs. In school, I remember being embarrassed as I would have to excuse myself from class until the coughing stopped. Often, the cold would turn serious with fevers and chills, and I would have to stay home from school. Though I was never sick enough to return to the hospital, I nevertheless suffered with these prolonged colds well into my thirties. I had figured that my lungs were weak and I was easily susceptible because of the pneumonia I had had as a child. I had learned to live with this infirmity all of these years. But God was about to show me another amazing piece to my healing.

> And, behold, there was a woman which had a spirit of infirmity eighteen years, and was bowed

> together, and could in no wise lift up herself. And when Jesus saw her, he called her to him, and said unto her, Woman, thou art loosed from thine infirmity. And he laid his hands on her: and immediately she was made straight, and glorified God.
>
> Luke 13:11–13 (KJV)

The Lord took me back to the time when I was seven when I had double pneumonia. He reminded me how the pneumonia had left me weak and frail. He revealed to me that during my illness, *a spirit of infirmity* attached itself to my lungs continuing to render me subject to debilitating colds. As the Lord revealed this to me, I was astonished at this insight. The word *infirmity* means "feebleness of body or mind, a malady, or frailty." It means "disease, sickness, or weakness." The root of the word infirmity in the Strong's Concordance means "without strength." In my weakened state as a child, Satan had taken advantage of me. He had moved in, so to speak, took up residence, and exerted his power and influence in this physical area of my body. When God shone his light on this, the spirit left immediately and I was free for quite some time. The spirits are subject to God, and when he reveals truth to us, the spirits can no longer stay. They can no longer pull the wool over our eyes. His truth will indeed set us free.

But here I was lying in bed, sick again, and this time, deathly sick. I could actually feel what little strength I had ebbing from my body. I was perplexed for I knew that God had healed me. As I weakly boxed the air with my fists, I suddenly *saw* Satan himself standing in the doorway to my bedroom. As he stood there, I could feel the heaviness of his thick black presence. I could sense his mocking stare as he stated with such certainty and finality, "I'm going to kill you!" he said.

As I continued declaring the Word of the Lord, "I shall live and not die!" the Lord spoke to me. "Forshia, you *are* healed. I *have* healed you. But Satan is trying with all of his might to open that door again. Don't believe him. Stand your ground." Indeed, as I resisted the lie, he eventually left and so did the symptoms. I would declare the works of the Lord!

Through this experience, I gained a very important and crucial understanding of healing. God heals, and he desires to heal. Satan steals, and he desires to steal. In John 10:10, Jesus says that Satan came to steal, kill, and destroy. Then Jesus says that he came that we might have life and have it to the full. Jesus came not only to give us life, but his desire is that we might experience life to the maximum possibility.

I also learned through this experience that it was my responsibility to resist Satan's lies. Just because God had healed me didn't mean that Satan would not try to steal my healing. I had always been easily swayed, but this experience was making me stronger. When Jesus was tempted in the wilderness by Satan, the Bible says that after he was tempted, Satan left until a more opportune time. This truth helped me see that Satan will try to come back to regain ground that we have already taken. I didn't have to be perplexed when this happened, but I needed to be aware, especially if I was in a weakened state of any kind. I learned to watch out.

Be self-controlled and alert. Your enemy the devil prowls around like a roaring lion looking for someone to devour. Resist him, standing firm in the faith, because you know that your brothers throughout the world are undergoing the same kind of sufferings. And the God of all grace, who called you to his eternal glory in Christ, after you have suffered a little while, will himself restore you and make you strong, firm and steadfast. To him be the power for ever and ever. Amen.

1 Peter 5:8–11

I was becoming strong. Praise God! I wanted to be strong. I didn't want to be so easily swayed every time I encountered a trial. Knowing my weaknesses did not keep God from being able to make me strong. I learned he could work with anyone. I was not a hopeless case, as I thought so many times. Who would have ever thought I could be a strong woman of faith? But God knew. To him is the power forever and ever. Amen! And yes, I often thought of those around the world who were going through the same kind of sufferings as I was. This gave me comfort. I wasn't alone. There was someone somewhere who was going through a similar trial, and they were winning. I could win too. I could be an example to others.

I began to view my trials differently. I began to see each victory as a stone being laid in the foundation of my temple. These stones were every kind of precious stones as spoken about in Revelation when Paul the apostle speaks of the New Jerusalem, the heavenly city.

THE WILDERNESS SHALL BLOSSOM LIKE THE ROSE

These stones would reflect the many-faceted grace of God. The gates of the city, the Bible says in Revelation, were one single pearl. I began to see that each weakness I overcame became like a single pearl. These pearls were replacing the gates or doors to my temple, my being.

Pearls—what a perfect symbol. Pearls are made through irritation. Pearls are made in the secret dark, quiet place of the shell. Pearls take time. Once, my mother-in-law had a pearl ring made for me for my birthday. She said she took quite a length of time to pick out a good pearl. I remember her telling me that her jeweler assured her that it was a fine pearl, having been in the shell for seven years. The pearl had a most wonderful sheen to it. It was beautiful. Yes, some things take time.

I began to see that God was rebuilding my life, my temple. Satan didn't have the last say. God did. Satan was subject to God and his Word. Satan stood at the door or gate of my weakness that day. His desire was to kill me. Through resisting him, he could not cross over the threshold. He stood, and I stood. He resisted, and I resisted. I found that when I resisted long enough, he had to flee. I won. I began to glory in my weaknesses. I saw that my weaknesses were an opportunity for Christ to live big in me. They were no longer my enemies. The Apostle Paul talks about this.

> But he said to me, "My grace is sufficient for you, for my power is made perfect in weakness." Therefore I will boast all the more gladly about my weaknesses, so that Christ's power may rest on me. That is why, for Christ's sake, I delight in

weaknesses, in insults, in hardships, in persecutions, in difficulties. For when I am weak, then I am strong.

> 2 Corinthians 12:9–10

How could I loose if even in weakness I was made strong?

When God told Moses to send some men into Canaan to check it out and bring back a report, he had in mind that they would be able to conquer the land and dwell there no matter the challenges. Indeed the land was a land flowing with milk and honey and the fruit bountiful. But the rest of their report was only negative. The people are powerful and of great size, they said, and the cities are fortified and very large. They spread a bad report among the Israelites and incited a riot, which did not please God. They said that they were like grasshoppers in their own eyes and that the inhabitants of the land viewed them the same also.

Only Joshua and Caleb saw it differently. Caleb insisted that they could take the land because God would be with them. But the people were afraid, and they rebelled against the Lord. Because of this, they did not enter Canaan. In fact, only Joshua and Caleb would enter the promised land along with the children of those who rebelled.

What I do appreciate about this true account is though the people rebelled, God forgave them. In fact, he forgave them time and time again. I always know that God will forgive me, but I have also learned there are consequences for *prolonged* disobedience. Succumbing to fear would keep me in the wilderness. I was determined to enter my promised land. I was determined to enter my Canaan. I was determined to stand and fight the good fight of faith. As I so often proclaim to myself, "I can do everything through him who gives me strength" (Philippians 4:13).

When Moses died, Joshua was chosen to lead the people that were left into the promised land. In preparation to enter, God told Joshua to be strong and courageous. He said he would be with him just as he was with Moses. He said he would never leave him nor forsake him. He emphasized it again: be strong and courageous for he would lead the people to inherit the land that was promised. And again, "Have I not commanded you? Be strong and courageous. Do not be terrified; do not be discouraged, for the Lord your God will be with you wherever you go" (Joshua 1:9). Then one more time, only this time it came from the people. A rallying cry of submission that they would do whatever Joshua commanded, only they encouraged him that he should be strong and courageous.

I love the fact that the people encouraged Joshua to be strong and courageous. More times than I can count, the body of Christ, my brothers and sisters in the Lord, would say to me in so many different ways, "Forshia, be strong and courageous." A phone call would come at just the right time or a card in the mail with just the right words. I kept a Hush Puppies shoebox under my bed containing all the cards, notes and letters that people sent me. I even had a McDonald's napkin in my shoebox that a woman from California mailed to me. The words written on it were just what I needed. I would often read my box full of "encouragement," and my spirits would soar. Joshua, Caleb, and the people inherited the land. So would I. I could see it! It was time to cross into the promised land—my promised land!

> And what more shall I say? I do not have time to tell about Gideon, Barak, Samson, Jephthah, David, Samuel and the prophets, who through faith conquered kingdoms, administered justice, and gained what was promised; who shut the mouths of lions, quenched the fury of the flames, and escaped the edge of the sword; whose weakness was turned to strength; and who became powerful in battle and routed foreign armies.
>
> Hebrews 11:32–34

A SPIRIT OF POVERTY

I fell prostrate on the bed, sobbing my eyes out. I couldn't do this anymore. It was too hard to put the lessons together. I didn't know what I was doing. God had called me to start a Bible study in my home. That in itself was amazing to me as I had no biblical training, had little confidence, and only a few attendees at the time. I sobbed uncontrollably. That day, I felt so defeated. Suddenly I felt a presence in my room. I slowly lifted my head and looked up. There before me stood a large six-foot creature covered in strips of rags from the top of his head to his feet. The rags were gray and soiled. Its eyes were large, dark and staring at me with a doleful, mournful, sorrowful look.

I jumped off of the bed and asked the Lord what it was. He said, "It is a spirit of poverty."

I began to rebuke the spirit in the name of Jesus. Nothing happened. I rebuked it again. Nothing happened. Finally, in desperation, I cried out to the Lord, "Why doesn't it leave?"

"Because," he said, "this is a spirit you need to overcome."

※

Up until this time, I had learned much about demonic influences and how to rebuke them. In actuality, it was simple. When the spirits are revealed, you simply tell them to go in the name of Jesus. Sometimes they would just go without a rebuke, as in the case of the spirit of infirmity I had struggled with. There didn't have to be an all-out hand-to-hand combat, as some of the movies portrayed. All through the Gospels, when Jesus encountered demonic spirits, he operated in full and calm authority. Jesus was my example, and he simply told them to go. At times, he would even forbid them to speak to him. This time though, it didn't work. As the Lord gave me more understanding, he showed me that this was a demonic stronghold that had a strong place in my thinking and therefore influenced my reactions and behavior toward certain pressures or challenges.

Poverty is an ugly thing. In fact, it is a curse. But being influenced by a poverty spirit is not just about the lack of money. Poverty can also be a state of mind. Its roots are imbedded in fear—fear of never having enough, fear that you can never succeed. It was the same with the Israelites. Each time a crisis appeared, they couldn't handle it. They grumbled and complained and rebelled, but in reality, it was about fear—fear that they couldn't overcome the challenge. Where there is fear, there can be no faith. Grumbling and complaining was simply a cover-up for the real issue. In their distress, they eluded to the fact that Egypt was a better place to be. Really? How can bondage be better?

Yes, the promised land had challenges. In fact, it was reported that there were giants in the land. Nevertheless, God had promised them the land, and he expected them to conquer it because he promised that his presence and power would be with them. He would see them through to the other side. Years and years of lack and failure in my past created in me a mind-set that I would not succeed. In order to overcome this poverty spirit, I would have to move forward. I could not succumb to my inadequacies. My fear of failure could not be the deciding factor.

> When a strong man, fully armed, guards his own house, his possessions are safe. But when someone stronger attacks and overpowers him, he takes away the armor in which the man trusted and divides up the spoils.
>
> Luke 11:21–22

The strong man in this scripture is Satan. As long as I had a mind-set with a bent toward failure, the strong man could hold my emotional house captive. In real life, when someone is taken hostage, it is because they are not strong enough or do not have the right weapons to resist the intrusion. Sometimes it is because of carelessness by not being aware of their surroundings. More often than not, there is more than one person involved in taking someone hostage. So it is in the kingdom of darkness. Satan has *cohorts* to help him execute his plot.

But God's plan was to redeem me. The word *redeem* is a wonderful word. It means "to buy back, to pay off, to carry out, to make good, to fulfill, to set free, to rescue, to save, to reclaim (land), to make up for, to balance, to regain, to liberate, to deliver, and to release." These all point to restoration and to God's redemptive plan not only for me but also for all of mankind. When Jesus died on the cross, he took my place. He did it right because I couldn't. He paid the price for all that I was incapable of doing and bought me back from the clutches of the enemy of my soul. He paid the ransom note. Hallelujah!

I was a threat to Satan's spiritual kingdom of darkness by allowing God to use me in teaching a Bible study. And the Bible study was growing as more people heard about it. Some of the women were even bringing their husbands. They thought the teachings were so good, they believed I should record them and put them on tape. After much prodding, I went to K-Mart and got a tape recorder, a lapel mic, and some blank tapes. After putting my teachings on tape, they offered to buy them. I was astonished at this. I remember when God first asked me to teach, I told him that I was no teacher. After all, I had never taught before. Who was I to teach others? But he had a different plan. Eventually, I started getting invitations to speak at churches. I learned that God loves to use the most unlikely candidates to show his power and accomplish his work.

Nevertheless, even though I was learning how to trust Jesus for strength to endure and continue to go

THE WILDERNESS SHALL BLOSSOM LIKE THE ROSE

forward, it still baffled me that the attacks of depression and suicide continued. Would I endure this battle forever? But another piece of the puzzle was about to be revealed. It would involve uncovering Satan's schemes.

Satan did not want my spiritual house to be in order. He didn't want Jesus to be King of my house. He did not want me to know that I had authority through Jesus Christ to disarm him, bind him, and tell him to leave me alone. Someone stronger than Satan has come on the scene. He has attacked and overpowered him, took away his armor, and is dividing up the spoils for all those who will receive it. This stronger man is Jesus Christ. He is the authentic one. He was getting ready to tie up this strong man so that I could be free from house arrest. "Or again, how can anyone enter a strong man's house and carry off his possessions unless he first ties up the strong man? Then he can rob his house" (Matthew 12:29). An incredible encounter was getting ready to take place in my life.

One day, a friend of mine introduced me to a couple from Texas. They were a quiet, unassuming couple full of love and gentleness. They began to tell me about their ministry of deliverance and how it could help me. A deliverance ministry is one by which a person, through the direction and power of the Holy Spirit, commands Satan to leave your soul area or your physical body. I shied away from deliverance ministries because I had heard that strange things happened during such events. I was afraid.

But God had his own plan for my healing, and He had a great surprise in store for me. It would be a day

I will never forget! Another dimension to my healing was about to take place. God was ready to tie up the strong man in my house so that I could be free and walk out my front door, lift my arms to heaven, my face toward the sun, and shout with abandonment, "I'm free, and the world is my oyster! I have found the pearl of great price, and it is Jesus."

> Praise be to the Lord my Rock, who trains my hands for war, my fingers for battle. He is my loving God and my fortress, my stronghold and my deliverer, my shield, in whom I take refuge, who subdues peoples under me.
>
> Psalm 144:1–2

This couple from Texas began to share with me that deliverance did not have to be bizarre. This was my fear. I had heard bizarre stories about deliverance. In the Bible, every time Jesus addressed Satan, Jesus was in control. He spoke boldly but confidently. And Satan was subdued in every instance. This couple shared with me the wonderful successful encounters they had had as God used them in this area to set people free. I began to feel peaceful about it. They made me feel safe, and I began to believe this was the answer I was looking for. I told the couple that I would like to go through this deliverance, and we set a time for this amazing encounter with God and these opposing forces in my life.

The first thing they challenged me to do after they opened the meeting with prayer was to have the Lord search my heart for any unforgiveness I might be harboring. I've learned since then that I cannot afford to harbor unforgiveness. If I hold unforgiveness in my life, Satan has a *reason* to take me hostage. "In your anger do not sin": Do not let the sun go down while you are still angry, and do not give the devil a foothold" (Ephesians 4:26–27).

There can be many reasons why Satan and his gang take a person hostage. Patterns of wrong behavior and attitudes are often passed down from one generation to another and become part of our spiritual DNA, just like physical problems can be passed down. These patterns had wreaked havoc in my life and the lives of others and became a place where Satan gained influence. Just as I had reaped the consequences of the sin of Adam and Eve, even though I did not eat the forbidden fruit, I was also reaping the consequences of the sins of my ancestors, parents, spouses, and unhealthy relationships. I also was reaping the consequences of my choices of the past. Negative experiences attract negative spirits. These patterns of behavior and attitudes become strongholds. A stronghold is anything that has a strong *hold* on you that is not God's best. Strongholds then give Satan a spiritually legal right to knock on your door. That's why it was imperative that I continue to renew my thinking according to God's truth—his Word.

When the deliverance session was over, the wife of the couple turned to me ever so gently and said, "See, that wasn't so hard." And it wasn't! She took me through a simple order of steps that revealed any areas that opened the door to these demonic strongholds. What amazed me was that she asked the Lord to search my heart. I was *not* to search my own heart. Because of my tendency to always feel responsible, this was a freeing step for me. After she prayed and asked for God's peace to be with us, she had me bow my head and *wait* for God's gentle impression concerning anyone I had not forgiven. I was encouraged when only one person came to mind as I had been trying diligently to follow the Lord's ways.

Then she asked the Lord to reveal any occult or witchcraft practices that I might have been involved with, past or present. I was surprised because I had been exposed to some things in my past that I had forgotten about. Once, I had someone read my fortune with tarot cards. I also used to read the horoscopes before I received the Lord into my life. I was then to ask God's forgiveness because these practices are an abomination to God because he does not want us tapping into any power but his. These demonic powers open the door to a dark realm. After this part was over, she then asked the Lord to show her any demonic spirits that had gained a foothold in my life. She named two spirits right away. They were spirits of *suicide* and *depression*. I actually felt and saw two entities leave the left side of my body immediately as she called them out. I was amazed.

As I look back over my life, many times I was in the wrong place at the wrong time. Standing at the bottom of the stairs so many years ago in the condemned house I tried to make a home, that spirit of depression visited me and moved in, and poverty came with it. Now I was no longer at the bottom. The promise of Deuteronomy 28:13 was coming to pass, "The Lord will make you the head, not the tail…you will always be at the top, never at the bottom." God was rebuilding my old house and making it brand new. He was refurnishing it with new stuff—the right stuff. I had made many wrong choices, but because I had made Jesus Christ the Lord of my life, he was reversing the effects of sin and the wrong choices that I had made. These choices had opened the door to demonic strongholds. He was cleaning out the skeletons in my family closet as there was a history in my family line of depression, emotional breakdowns, and poverty. I was going to have a fresh start.

When our session was all finished, the lady from Texas said that these spirits were bound and the Lord would cause them to stay away as he helped me master new habits of thinking and right attitudes about myself. Satan would have no place in me as these areas became filled up with the right things, godly things.

Then her husband said one more thing. He said, "I bind a spirit of Alzheimer that will try to visit her in years to come." And so it did some twenty years later, and I resisted it, and it left me alone. Praise his holy name! This was by no means the answer for all problems in my life. Not every problem has a demon behind it. It would take wisdom from God and listening continually to his voice to decipher the solutions to life's issues. But this was a major turning point in my healing. Jesus is the deliverer. Praise his holy name.

And so all Israel will be saved, as it is written: "The deliverer will come from Zion; he will turn godlessness away from Jacob. And this is my covenant with them when I take away their sins."

Romans 11:26–27

WHAT ABOUT MY CHILDREN?

I gripped the steering wheel and started to cry uncontrollably. I couldn't take it anymore. My husband and I were having so many problems with my daughter, Tiffany. Skipping school, coming in late at night, and hanging with the wrong crowd were just a few. Now she was in trouble with the law and was having to submit to counseling and probation through the legal system. No matter what my husband and I did, she rebelled. I didn't know what else to do. My prayers seemed fruitless. What is going to happen to my daughter? Suddenly, a peace came over me, and the Lord spoke strongly to me, *Forshia, I'm going to take care of your daughter. Not because she deserves it but because I have made a covenant with you!*

> He is the Lord our God; His judgments are in all the earth. He is (earnestly) mindful of His covenant *and* forever it is imprinted on His

heart, the word which He commanded *and* established to a thousand generations…

Psalm 105:7-8 (AMP)

Tiffany and I practically grew up together. I was only nineteen when she was born—a child having a child. It broke my heart when Wayne brought a bouquet of pink flowers to the hospital with tiny blue ones sprinkled throughout. He said he just wanted to make sure that I knew he had wanted a boy. How cruel! He was a cruel man. His rejection of Tiffany was a rejection of me. I wouldn't realize until I became a Christian that the effect of this rejection from Tiffany's father would carry through to her adult years. She would struggle in searching for a father's love, just as I did. My countless unhealthy relationships with men would take its toll on my daughter. I remember vividly one time when I broke an engagement to be married to a man that truly loved Tiffany. She was only five years old. I remember her crying and exclaiming, "Mommy, he promised to be my daddy." Yet the reason I broke up with him was because he was an alcoholic too, just like her real father, Wayne. I seemed to be drawn to the *bad boy* types. But all my daughter knew was that another father figure was being ripped from her life. Moving from pillar to post, relationship-to-relationship created an emotional instability in the both of us that left its mark. Yet we were close, just like sisters sometimes. I didn't always make mature decisions. One time I remember buying a big box of malt balls because we loved malt balls. We ate the whole box together and got sick. To this day she

THE WILDERNESS SHALL BLOSSOM LIKE THE ROSE

says she has a love-hate relationship with malt balls. I didn't always shield her, as I should have. I didn't always do the right thing, but I loved her.

At the time I was married to my second husband, Bill, we were living in Mobile, Alabama. Bill loved Tiffany. To this day, Tiffany still comments on how she knew that he really loved her. She still remembers the beautiful dress he bought for her one time. But his drug addiction destroyed everything. After the divorce I moved back to Montgomery and began working for the Veterans Administration again. I had had a good job with them before I had married Bill. With the tumultuous marriage ended, I yearned for stability. I wanted a normal life. So I rented a cute little house and made a commitment to myself never to do drugs again and try to make up for all the turmoil I had put Tiffany through. I even reserved Sundays to be with her. I determined not to let anything interfere with that day. Why Sunday? It could have been Saturday, but I think subconsciously I was trying to appease God for the guilt I felt.

Sundays were always hard for me. I couldn't put my finger on why but there was a lonely feeling about Sundays. I remember feeling different and left out when I would take my daughter out to lunch on Sundays. I would see other families all dressed up in their Sunday best with complete families, a mother, father, and children. I wanted to be like them. I yearned for a normal family life. There would be times when I would try to go to church. But we didn't seem to fit in. I was a single mom and didn't fit in with the adult Sunday school class because everyone was married. I didn't fit in with the single's Sunday school class because no one was divorced. Their issues seemed shallow and minor compared to mine. I just didn't fit.

One day Tiffany was invited to go to a neighborhood Vacation Bible School. I didn't want to have anything to do with it but allowed the church bus to pick her up each day and drop her off. Each time the school bus driver stopped to pick her up, he would lean his head out the door and ask me to come with them. I always answered an irritated *no* as I puffed away on my cigarette. The last day of VBS, she stepped off from the school bus beaming. I asked her how things went. She proceeded to tell me how she had asked Jesus into her heart and how excited she was. "Jesus loves me," she said. I promptly told her that it wasn't real and I didn't believe in that kind of stuff and she shouldn't either. I remember the disappointment in her eyes. I crushed her excitement. She was around six years old.

Not so soon after that, I met Eric. When he asked me for a date to go to the drive-in, it would be on a Sunday. I told him plainly that I kept that day reserved to spend with my daughter. He quickly answered, "Bring her along." I was surprised as most of the men I dated didn't want to *bring* her along. After we married, within days Tiffany was telling her friends that Eric was her new dad. She was so proud. But we all struggled in the coming months with our new family. Eric had never been a father before, and I fought him on some of the ways he wanted to parent her. I came with much emotional baggage and was possessive of how Tiffany was to be parented. Needless to say, Eric and I clashed more often than not.

Within a matter of months, Eric received orders for Tinker AFB in Oklahoma City, Oklahoma, in August of 1976. Our son, Dax, would be born the following summer and with his arrival, a new set of conflicting circumstances and emotions would begin to stir within our family. Tiffany felt left out and she struggled with feelings of rejection. I felt in the middle trying to hold it all together. This was my third marriage, and for a third time, I would begin to look for a way out. But God had another plan in mind. A spiritual intervention of monumental proportions would catapult me into a new life and cause me to recommit to the marriage. I was attending the University of Oklahoma at the time and had just finished the spring session when I was introduced to the Gospel and committed my life to Jesus. Immediately, the Lord instructed me not to go back to school. He wanted me to devote my time and energies to being a wife and mother. I had a lot to make up for. Within weeks I would find a church and begin to take my children. God saw to it that we fit in. We were received with open arms. Though my husband did not receive the Lord for many years, I would pray for my children consistently and teach them about God. Around the age of twelve, Tiffany refused to go to church anymore. She was struggling with the inner turmoil of the family. I was mortified when she told me she put God in a jar and put him on the shelf. The last time that I remember her going to church she stood during worship with a scowl on her face and her arms folded in defiance. I grieved. I felt I had lost her.

I know God must have felt that way when the Israelites would stray away from him. It must have broken his heart. I can almost hear him thinking. *If they only knew how much I love them. If they only knew I only want to do them good. Don't they know I am always here for them?* Every time the Israelites got into trouble and cried out to the Lord for help, he rescued them. *Don't they know I am faithful and can be trusted?* "It will also come to pass that before they call, I will answer; and while they are still speaking, I will hear" Isaiah 65:24 (NASB). He would continue to love her, seek her, and take care of her. He wouldn't give up on her.

One day, during those turbulent, challenging teenage years my daughter ran away from home. The next day the doorbell rang. I opened the front door to see a young man standing on my steps. The young teenage boy's words were jolting. "Mrs. Ross, you don't know me, but I just wanted to tell you that your daughter is okay. I can't tell you where she is, but I just wanted you to know." Then he took off running. Closing the front door, I turned around and stood with my back to the door and began to shake. *Where is she?* Immediately, a scripture came to me from Isaiah 65:23. "They will not labor in vain, Or bear *children* for calamity; For they are the offspring of those blessed by the LORD, And their descendants with them" (NASB). I chose to believe it. I chose to trust that God's Word was true and he would take care of her. Three days later she came home. Test after test came concerning my daughter. I chose to

THE WILDERNESS SHALL BLOSSOM LIKE THE ROSE

continue to pray and believe that the Lord was faithful. Despite everything, Tiffany graduated from high school a year early, worked full time, and paid her father back in three months for a car he bought for her. She was always a hard worker.

When Tiffany left home at eighteen and married a marine, I missed her terribly, but I continued to pray for her and her new husband. At the time, her husband was stationed at Camp Lejeune in North Carolina. When Tiffany became pregnant, their financial situation took a turn for the worse. I began to pray. Early in the morning I would rise and petition the Lord and remind him how he had told me that my children had not been created for calamity—how he said he would take care of her, not because she deserved it, but because he had made a covenant with me. In those early hours one morning I read Psalm 37:25, "I was young and now I am old, yet I have never seen the righteous forsaken or their children begging bread." Because I was righteous, I could claim this scripture. I was right before God and yet, even in that, I was only righteous based upon my trust in him and what he had done for me when he died on the cross for my sins.

> God made him who had no sin to be sin for us, so that in him we might become the righteousness of God.
>
> 2 Corinthians 5:21

> For in the gospel a righteousness from God is revealed, a righteousness that is by faith from

first to last, just as it is written: "The righteous will live by faith."

            Romans 1:17

 This journey with my children would have to be a walk of faith, not based on what I saw but based upon God's trustworthiness. He had made a covenant with me, and he would keep his end of the bargain no matter how long it took. My faith would be tested many times in years to come, not only with my daughter, but with my son also. I wanted more than anything for my children to experience the joy I had in knowing the Lord. I would learn many things through the years as I prayed for my children and sought the Lord on their behalf. Some of the things I learned had to do with breaking negative generational curses in their lives through prayer. Some had to do with allowing my children to come back to the Lord in their own time. Some simply had to do with enjoying them for who they were and not what I wanted them to become. Some of the things I learned even had to do with me going on with my own life and following the Lord. God was calling me into ministry, and he was calling me right in the middle of it all. I learned not to fret or be anxious, not to lose sleep or give up and not to turn away from the Lord when it looked like nothing would change. Don't get me wrong. I'll always be a mom, and I'll always have opportunity to be concerned for them. But most of all, I have learned that God loves my children *more* than I do.

Twenty years and four children later, Tiffany left her marriage. It had been a very difficult one. It was a painful time for her. During this time, Tiffany confronted me on some things that she had kept inside. It was a painful time for me but necessary. She is now married to her childhood sweetheart. They are very happy. How's her spiritual progress? Well, I'm still praying and sometimes we pray over the phone and text a lot. And we laugh a lot. In fact when I inquired of her for permission to write this chapter, she swears that all her stepdad and I did during those years was ground her every other day. It's probably almost true. We're still growing together and learning from each other. I remember vividly one time when we were having dinner and Tiffany said something disrespectful to me. I flipped out, reached across the table, grabbed her by the collar, and without missing a beat, practically dragged Tiffany upstairs. I had had it. Mild mannered me had lost it. I remember Eric and Dax's eyes were as big as saucers as they stared at each other with forks in midair. They had never seen me like this. It's funny now. I'm glad we can laugh about it. Tiffany is an amazing woman, a strong woman. She's creative like me. She's persevering and smart and spontaneously funny too.

I'll always remember these pivotal words from the Lord, "Forshia, I'm going to take care of your daughter. Not because she deserves it but because I've made a covenant with you!" Now, I hear these words a bit more fully. "Forshia, I'm going to take care of your daughter, your son, your grandchildren, and one day your great-grandchildren down to a thousand generations! Why?

Because I've made a covenant with you!" Wow! Our God is an awesome God. What a statement he made to me. I know now the Lord was saying that his ability to straighten out our children is not dependant on how they are acting, or how rebellious they are toward him or any of those things. It is strictly based on his promise He made with me—his relationship with me. During the difficult years of Tiffany's marriage, she took her children to church–alone–regularly. There is a promise from God concerning our children that I love. "Train up a child in the way he should go: and when he is old, he will not depart from it" (Proverbs 22:6, KJV). I've claimed that promise. I claim that promise for my grandchildren. Moms rock! Listen to this,

> For when God made (His) promise to Abraham, He swore by himself, since He had no one greater by whom to swear…
>
> This was so that, by two unchangeable things (His promise and His oath) in which it is impossible for God ever to prove false or deceive us…
>
> Hebrews 6:13, 18 (AMP)

What is a covenant? It is a solemn or binding agreement either written or promised between two or more parties. His covenant or promise concerning our children is based, not on our feelings or how they are acting, but on God's faithfulness to his promise. He has settled the matter. Why, it's just a matter of time. Isn't that a relief?

THE WILDERNESS SHALL BLOSSOM LIKE THE ROSE

> Do not be afraid, for I am with you; I will bring your children from the east and gather you from the west. I will say to the north, 'Give them up!' and to the south, 'Do not hold them back.' Bring my sons from afar and my daughters from the ends of the earth—
>
> Isaiah 43:5-6

ROSES, ROSES, EVERYWHERE ROSES

*E*ric got out of the car and stood before me holding one half dozen red roses in his hand. He had come to take Tiffany and me to the movies. I was flabbergasted.

"Why are you bringing me roses?" I asked. We had just met the night before. *He does not know me well enough to bring me roses*, I was thinking.

"You have the saddest eyes I have ever seen," he said. "I thought these might cheer you up."

The roses made a huge impact on me. And yes, I knew my eyes were sad. In fact, I would look into the mirror quite often and smile at myself, trying to make my smile reach my eyes, but it never did. My eyes never lit up anymore. Little did I know that the half dozen red roses would be a sign and an installment on the future work that God would do in my life. I didn't know, but God knew.

Everywhere I looked, there were roses. I had never noticed them before. Even in the pattern of my bedspread. There were roses in the plates I had just bought. There were roses in my living and dinning-room curtains. They were all over the house in one form or another. I was also reminded about the time when I was seven years old when I tried my hand at oil painting. My first painting was of a rose in full bloom. My grandmother loved it so much she hung it in her bedroom. In that same year, I would be chosen queen to represent my first grade. This was a big deal. Each grade chose a king and queen during the Christmas season. The dress was formal, and all candidates would be present on stage, as the winner would be announced. The Lord reminded me how my mother made me a beautiful white crinoline gown with tiny rosebuds sewn to the waist. I remember my mother and I had gone to town to look for shoes to match the gown and how awed we were when we discovered black patent leather shoes with tiny red rosebuds attached to the neck of the shoes. Yes, roses, roses, everywhere roses.

The most amazing discovery of roses was in the blouse I had just bought. I was still struggling with my weight, and I desperately wanted to have victory in this area. When I saw the blouse in the store, I fell in love with it immediately. It had a huge collar that draped slightly over the shoulders with delicately wrought embroidery work of flowers and roses throughout the fabric. The fabric was made of tissue faille. It was beautiful but very expensive. The only size that was left was the size I wore when I was at my right weight. I felt so strongly that the Lord wanted me to buy it anyway. I bought it and hung it in my closet. Sometimes, I would get it out and look at it.

When I went into the mental ward years before, I was underweight and couldn't eat, but within a matter of months, my weight ballooned up to nearly two hundred pounds due to powerful antidepressant medicines that were given to me. My depression had been put into check by these medicines, and I was thankful for them, but my weight was like a runaway train. No matter how hard I tried, I couldn't seem to loose the weight. Attending the Kay Arthur Bible study during that time had begun to help give me hope that God had answers for every area of my life.

One day, as I was crying out to the Lord about this problem, he impressed upon me that he would show me how to loose the weight. The answer turned out to be very simple. Every time I sat down to eat, he would whisper to me, "Forshia, that's enough now. Don't eat any more." As I continued to listen to his voice concerning how much to eat, the weight began to melt off. Within a matter of some six months, I had lost all of the extra weight. The women in the Bible study marveled as they saw me being transformed before their eyes.

But maintaining the weight loss was proving to be a different matter altogether. My weight occupied far too much of my thinking and was beginning to contribute to old feelings of failure. Here I was again, several years later, slipping back into old eating habits and struggling with ten to fifteen pounds of extra weight. Eventually, the Lord led me to join Weight Watchers. I had tried every weight loss program on the market up until then. I would loose the ten to fifteen pounds but gain it all back again. I lost the excess weight again on Weight Watchers and planned on quitting, but God had another plan in mind. I found it was always easier to loose than maintain. The Lord made it clear that I needed to go through their maintenance program.

In so doing, I became a lifetime member and took a part-time job there for a while. I really enjoyed it. Interestingly enough, the Lord did not open up the Bible study in my home until after this last piece of my healing was in place.

I remember standing in my bedroom one day when this thought came to me from the Lord. I had been questioning myself about why I had so much trouble with this weight thing. The thought was, "Forshia, what you need is discipline."

"Discipline!" I said out loud. "I know that. Of course, I need discipline. I just don't have any."

"You're right, you don't," said the Lord. "But I do. Draw upon my discipline. Remember, I reside within you. Draw upon my power."

Wow! I had never seen it like that before. I could maintain because I *did* have discipline, God's discipline within me. I could apply self-discipline to everything. I could choose to obey the Word of God in every situation.

> But the fruit of the Spirit is love, joy, peace, patience, kindness, goodness, faithfulness, gentleness and self-control. Against such things there is no law.
>
> Galatians 5:22-23

I would have many opportunities over the years to exercise this fruit. When I did, it was always there. Maintenance would prove to be an important key to my spiritual growth and stability. Just like cars or houses or relationships break down when they are not maintained, so could my body, soul and spirit if I did not maintain what God has done for me.

In preparation for entering the promised land, God reminded the Israelites of all that he had done for them—how they were tested to reveal what was in their hearts, how he had caused them to hunger and then fed them with manna to teach them that man does not live by bread alone but by every word that comes from the mouth of the Lord, how their clothes did not wear out. He told them, "Know then in your heart that as a man disciplines his son, so the Lord your God disciplines you" (Deuteronomy 8:5). He reminded them of all of this, so that when they reaped the promises, they would not forget.

> When you have eaten and are satisfied, praise the Lord your God for the good land he has given you. Be careful that you do not forget the Lord your God, failing to observe his commands, his laws and his decrees that I am giving you this day.
>
> Deuteronomy 8:10–11

One day, I was lying on the couch discouraged. My discouragement turned to tears as I cried over some other struggles I was having. It wasn't so much that I wasn't gaining victory over these struggles and not endeavoring to trust the Lord, but sometimes it was just plain hard to push through. Sometimes, I just wanted to lie down on the couch and not have to get up. This was such a day. Suddenly, the Lord spoke to my heart with these words, "Forshia, one day you will write a book and the book will be called *No Secondhand Rose, My Name is Forshia*. It will be the first of a trilogy about your journey to wholeness."

Did I hear right? I thought. *I don't know how to write a book.* It would be fourteen years before I would be able to write my first book, which was published in the year 2000. As the years rolled by, many times I thought that maybe it was all in my head and the Lord didn't say this at all. Sometimes I would share this promise with the wrong people, and they would discourage me. Sometimes I would try to sit down and write the book, but the words wouldn't come. So I waited and waited and continued to move forward. The scripture in Isaiah 40:31 became a scripture that I lived by, "But they that wait upon the LORD shall renew their strength; they shall mount up with wings as eagles; they shall run, and not be weary; and they shall walk, and not faint" (KJV).

As I waited, the speaking engagements started coming and the teachings on tape grew into a library and my ministry grew. I would begin to be invited to speak at different denominations. I would be asked to do conferences, seminars, and workshops. It was an incredible thing that unfolded as I trusted the Lord. God would even open up radio and television to me. Using the skills I had learned through the Kay Arthur Bible study that had so changed my life, I would even create a workbook called, *How I Overcame Depression and You Can, Too* and hold workshops. People would be encouraged and healed in these workshops and given tools to help them overcome. Once when I held one of these workshops, everyone that attended came in with sad faces but by lunchtime everyone's countenance had changed for the better. They were amazed at how studying the truth in God's Word could bring change so quickly. One time I received an e-mail from a pastor in Ghana, West Africa, that was so encouraged by my teachings on my website, treasuresfromtheheart.org, that he printed every page of my website and shared them with his church. One time I prayed for a man that had suffered with the fear of germs since he was five. He was healed and tells how after he went home he was able to touch everything in his house without fear. People would share over the years how they would experience healing in their minds, their bodies and their hearts through the different aspects of my ministry. But at the time I was lying on the couch, I did not know any of this would take place in the future.

I got up off the couch and dried my eyes. God knew best, of course. His timing was perfect. I couldn't imagine how all that he had told me would come to pass. I went upstairs and stood before the mirror, pondering the long journey I had made up until then. Thanking him for the weight loss, I reached into the closet and took out the beautiful blouse with the embroidered roses and slipped it on. It fit perfectly. It was amazing how he had prompted me to buy it *before* I could fit into it. Promises are like that. "For the revelation awaits an appointed time; it speaks of the end and will not prove false. Though it linger, wait for it; it will certainly come and will not delay" (Habakkuk 2:3). As the Israelites moved through the wilderness, God promised them the Promised Land. Thank you, Lord. I praise you. You have done so much for me.

 I had a dream once that I was speaking and standing on a high stage. After I finished speaking I invited people in the audience to come forward for ministry. One woman who had come forward exclaimed with an excited voice, "I smell roses!" My feet were about eye level to her. I leaned over and answered her, "That means healing." Over the years my book *No Secondhand Rose* has ministered healing to countless people. I don't know if anyone has "smelled" roses when they have read it, but I do know that countless people have been healed through it, both men and women. Once I had a women tell me that one sentence in the book had healed her from a broken relationship with her mother. Once I donated *No Secondhand Rose* to a men's prison. I remember at the time that I wondered why the Lord would want me to give it to a men's prison. After all, the front cover had a rose on it. A year later around Christmas time I received a letter from an inmate in that prison. He shared how of all the books in the library he had to choose from, he felt to choose mine. When he read my book, he said he was instantly delivered from depression. He had been very depressed since coming to prison. He also shared how he accepted the invitation at the back of the book to receive Jesus as his Lord and Savior. His name is Ernesto, and he was thrilled. I

THE WILDERNESS SHALL BLOSSOM LIKE THE ROSE

later called the prison chaplain, and the chaplain said Ernesto was a changed person.

Outside of my office window is a rose of Sharon bush. I love it. But for some reason, though it was in a good location, it had had difficulty flourishing in the first few years after my husband planted it for me. But now it was doing well. It made it, and so did I. During the summer, I love to stop, take a breather from my work, and look at it. Sometimes I count the blossoms. Each summer there is an increase. I also think back fondly to the time when I was a little girl and my mother would make me dolls out of the blossoms and buds using toothpicks. The rose of Sharon was a bright spot in my life.

> The wilderness and the solitary place shall be glad for them; and the desert shall rejoice, and blossom as the rose. It shall blossom abundantly, and rejoice even with joy and singing: the glory of Lebanon shall be given unto it, the excellency of Carmel and Sharon, they shall see the glory of the LORD, and the excellency of our God.
>
> Isaiah 35:1–2 (KJV)

Jesus has been called the Rose of Sharon. In Song of Songs 2:1–2, the scriptures read, "I am a rose of Sharon, a lily of the valleys. Like a lily among thorns is my darling among the maidens." He makes up for the thorns in our life. He walks us through the valleys. We don't have to stay there. There is a song we sing in church sometimes, and one of the lines expresses that he was like a rose trampled on the ground when he died on the cross. The song goes on to say that he was thinking of me when he took the fall.

He was thinking of all of mankind when he died on the cross. When he *rose* again his offer to us was a new life for all who trust him.

Many, many years later, on one my birthdays, my husband came home with roses—red roses. Interestingly though, it would only be one-half dozen. At first I wondered why I never received a dozen red roses. *Shouldn't they be a dozen? Isn't there something written somewhere about that?* I thought.

But God knew what he was doing as he whispered in my ear, "This, my dear one, is the rest of the installment on my promise. You are no secondhand rose."

> I am coming soon. Hold on to what you have, so that no one will take your crown. Him who overcomes I will make a pillar in the temple of my God. Never again will he leave it. I will write on him the name of my God and the name of the city of my God, the new Jerusalem, which is coming down out of heaven from my God; and I will also write on him my new name. He who has an ear, let him hear what the Spirit says to the churches.
>
> Revelation 3:11–13

EPILOGUE

As I prepare to send this manuscript to the publisher, I am overcome with laughter at myself. Here I am, having to put down on paper the tremendous trials and tribulations of my life and how I overcame them through obedience and trusting the Lord, and I am struggling right now with a big issue of obedience. This is too funny! The big difference now is that I used to fall into deep guilt, condemnation, and depression over struggling in obeying the Lord. I wanted to be perfect. I wanted to please God. In fact, I tried so hard at times I felt as if I would burst at the seams from straining. Honestly!

Don't get me wrong. I don't take *not* obeying the Lord lightly. I understand the consequences. But now I understand that the ultimate purpose of Satan in using guilt and condemnation is to keep us from relying on God's power to obey. I also understand that God does not throw us out when we fail to obey. You see, I believe guilt gives sin its power. Guilt cripples and deforms our ability to understand that it is God's power that we must rely upon to give us victory, not ours. Satan would want to say to me, even now, "Who are you to encourage people to yield to God if you are struggling?" But I do recognize that voice, and I do recognize that guilt is one of the most powerful means the enemy will use to keep my mouth shut and yours.

But it doesn't work anymore or at least not for long. I *will* share and I *will* declare the wondrous works of the redemptive power of God. In fact, I will shout it from the rooftops! And I will obey because God redeemed us that we might be able to trust him and yield to him because he loves us. In obedience, there are great blessings! Some beyond our wildest dreams! And so, know this, my dear ones. As long as we are in these flesh suits, there will be opportunities to make decisions to obey God, and the better we get at choosing God's way, the more cunning and subtle our enemy becomes in weaving plausible arguments to the contrary.

As I have shared in this book, one of the greatest truths that I learned that was a pivotal turning point in my journey to wholeness was in Romans 8:1–2 which says, "Therefore, there is now no condemnation for those who are in Christ Jesus, because through Christ Jesus the law of the Spirit of life set me free from the law of sin and death." When I couldn't seem to get it right, I learned that I was not condemned even as I was struggling to obey—even when I failed. I was in Christ Jesus, and He was in me. I was not guilty by reason of faith in His finished work. This caused me to continue to look to Jesus for my deliverance.

Think about it. If I could somehow accomplish the ability to overcome, then who would get the credit?

Ultimately the credit goes to God, who provided a way for us to obey. These struggles always remind me of my need for Him. After all, does not the Apostle Paul say in Romans 7:24–25, "What a wretched man I am! Who will rescue me from this body of death? Thanks be to God—through Jesus Christ our Lord!" What a wretched woman I was, but *he* rescued me. *He* set me free.

I am reminded of a dream I had in the early years of my healing. In the dream, I was in a country store with my sister. We were probably around ten and six respectively. I believe we were there to buy penny candy. It was summer, and we each had on matching shorts and a halter top that my mother had made for us, and of course, we were barefoot. Southerners go barefoot in the summer. In the dream, I was looking at us from above as an adult. Then I reached down and hugged myself as a little girl really hard and woke up. "What does this mean, Lord?" I asked.

He showed me that I was going to have to learn to love myself, accept myself, and embrace who I was. In doing this, the rejected little girl in me would be healed and would grow up. This took many years as I asked the Lord to teach me about his love. One day, I remember actually feeling his tangible embrace around me. God is love, and Jesus is the essence of his love.

Jesus tells us about love in Matthew 22:37-38. The Jewish teachers had asked Jesus which was the greatest commandment in the Law. Jesus's reply was this, "Love the Lord your God with all your heart and with all your soul and with all your mind. This is the first and greatest commandment." And then he said that the second was like it. "Love your neighbor as yourself" (Matthew 22:39).

I did learn to love myself. I began to see myself obedient, healed, and full of God. Through this, all the rejection I had experienced in my life began to be healed. What mercy the Father has bestowed upon us that we might be called the sons and daughters of God.

May you accept yourself as God has made you. May you begin to see yourself loved, obedient, healed, and full of the living God. May you be filled with courage to believe that he can use you, deliver you, and make you whole. This is the gospel. This is the good news.

Excuse me for just a moment. The phone is ringing. "Hello," I answer. "Yes, this is Forshia Ross… Yes, I am available on that date… Yes, I can speak to your group… The message? Well, I believe the message title is going to be Do You Need a New Beginning?"

You may not be able to come to hear my message, but you can have a new beginning in your life right now. John 3:16 says, "For God so loved the world that he gave his one and only Son, that whoever believes in him shall not perish but have eternal life."

Pray with me.

> Jesus, I believe God the Father sent you to this earth. I believe that you died on the cross and were buried and on the third day, you rose again.

THE WILDERNESS SHALL BLOSSOM LIKE THE ROSE

Come into my heart and forgive me of all my sins. I want to experience your love. Help me to start over. Heal me and give me peace, hope and purpose. Amen!